The yoga postures (asanas) described and illustrated in this book require the use of specific musical elixirs that are included with the purchase of this book. The elixirs work in conjunction with the postures, using the alchemical potencies of frequency incorporated within them.

• To download the music, go to: www.yogaofillumination.com

# ARANASH SUBA YOGA

## The Yoga of Enlightenment

Almine

Published by Spiritual Journeys LLC

First edition December 2012

Copyright 2012

MAB 998 Megatrust

By Almine
Spiritual Journeys LLC
P.O. Box 300
Newport, Oregon 97365

US toll-free phone: 1-877-552-5646

www.spiritualjourneys.com

All rights reserved. No part of this publication may be reproduced without written permission of the publishers.

Cover Illustration by Dorian Dyer
www.visionheartart.com

Manufactured in the United States of America

ISBN 978-1-936926-50-3 Softcover

ISBN 978-1-936926-51-0 Adobe reader

# Table of Contents

*Endorsements* ........................................................................... xi
*About the Author* ................................................................... xiii
*Liability Disclaimer* ................................................................ xv

Introduction to Aranash Suba Yoga ............................................. 1
How to do the Yoga .................................................................... 3
Becoming the Contradiction ....................................................... 6
Dancing with the Contradiction ................................................. 7

**Part I**
The Yoga Postures .................................................................... 11

**Part II**
Insights into the Eternal Dance From the Scrolls of Hanasat ....... 51

**Part III**
Related Insights from the Tablets of Gogekli Tepe
Secrets from the Whale Libraries .............................................. 71

**Closing** .................................................................................. 91

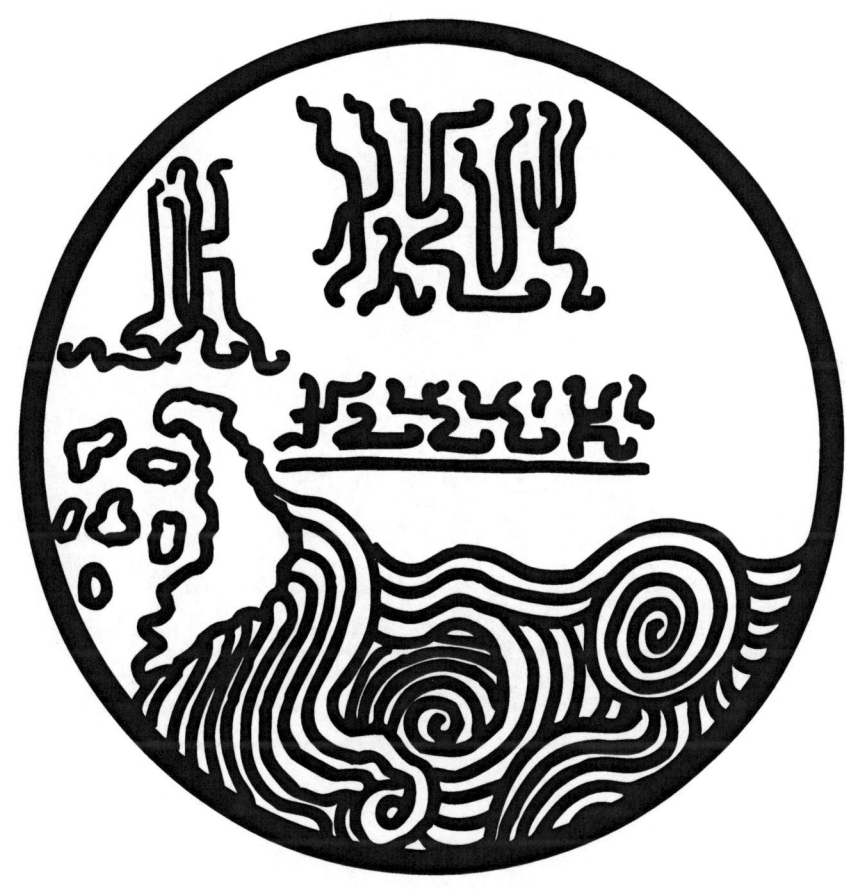

Aranash Suba Yoga

The Yoga of Enlightenment

# Endorsements

"What a priceless experience to be able to catch a glimpse into one of the most remarkable lives of our time…"

H.E. Ambassador Armen Sarkissian,
Former Prime Minister of the Republic of Armenia,
Astrophysicist, Cambridge University, U.K.

"I'm really impressed with Almine and the integrity of her revelations. My respect for her is immense and I hope that others will find as much value in her teaching as I have."

Dr. Fred Bell, Former NASA Scientist
Author of *The Promise*

"The information she delivers to humanity is of the highest clarity. She is fully deserving of her reputation as the leading mystic of our age."

Zbigniew Ostas, Ph.D. Quantum Medicine,
Somatidian Orthobiology, Canada and Poland

# About the Author

Almine is widely regarded as the leading mystic of our time and is the author of more than 30 books that have been translated into 11 languages. She is the originator of the globally acclaimed healing modality, Belvaspata, and shares her wisdom daily with a rapidly growing worldwide audience. (See www.alminediary.com, www.facebook.com/SeersWisdom and www.twitter.com/alminewisdom.) Her profound wisdom and unparalleled interdimensional abilities have been acclaimed by scientists and students alike.

*When we live in the moment, we live in the place of power,*
*aligned with eternal time and the intent of the Infinite.*
*Our will becomes blended with that of the Divine.*

Almine

# Liability Disclaimer

Any liability, loss, damage or injury in connection with the use of Aranash Suba Yoga and its instruction, included but not limited to any performance of the yoga, is expressly disclaimed by Spiritual Journeys, LLC and/or Almine.

Many have subluxations and misalignments in the neck and or spine. The postures involving the neck and spine should be done gently and with care not to strain these areas. Seeking chiropractic treatment prior to attempting this yoga may be beneficial.

Yoga is not intended to diagnose illness or to constitute medical advice or treatment. All persons with a medical condition, (including pregnancy) or any other health-related condition that may affect performance of the yoga, are advised to consult with a physician or other qualified health provider prior to its use in order to obtain medical approval to participate in the yoga.

# Interdimensional Photo of An Angel Sitting on Almine's Shoulder as She Sings

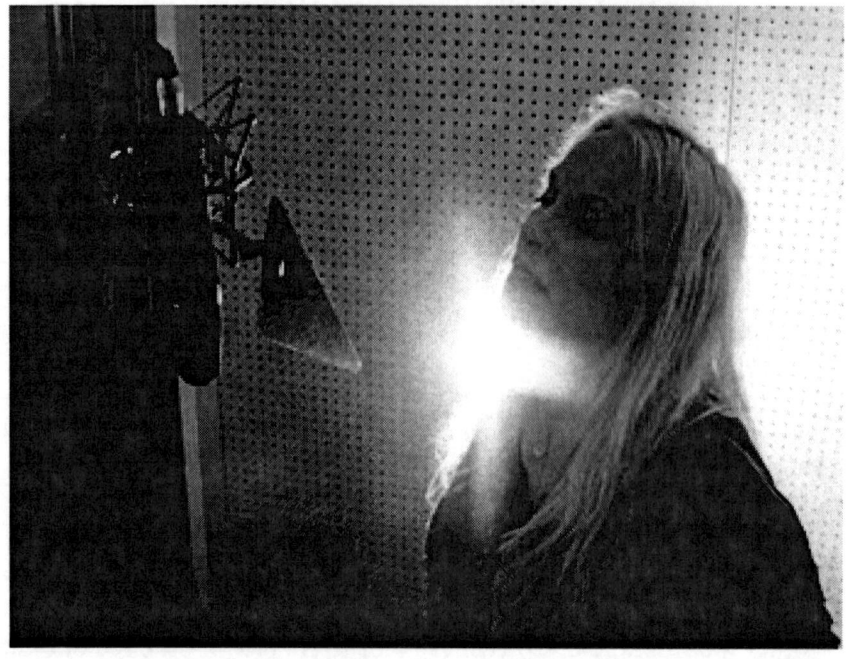

Photo taken in Almine's recording studio

Both the vocal and the instrumental components for Aranash Suba Yoga were received and performed in 2 hours.

# Interdimensional Photo of Almine Writing about Aranash Suba Yoga

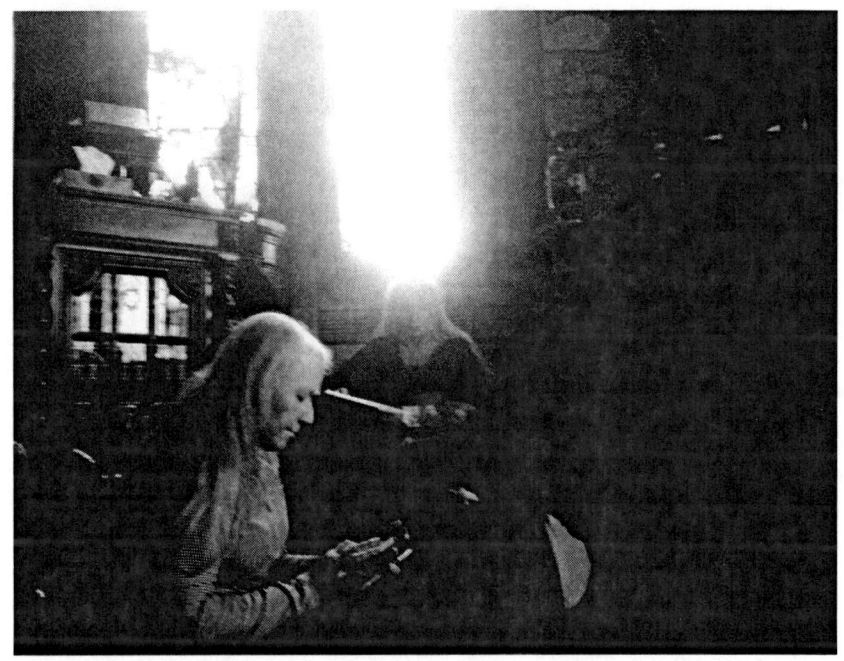

Photo taken by Donna, Canada

In this photo, Almine is writing a message for the person beside her as to how the book should be compiled; note the energy coming out of her pen.

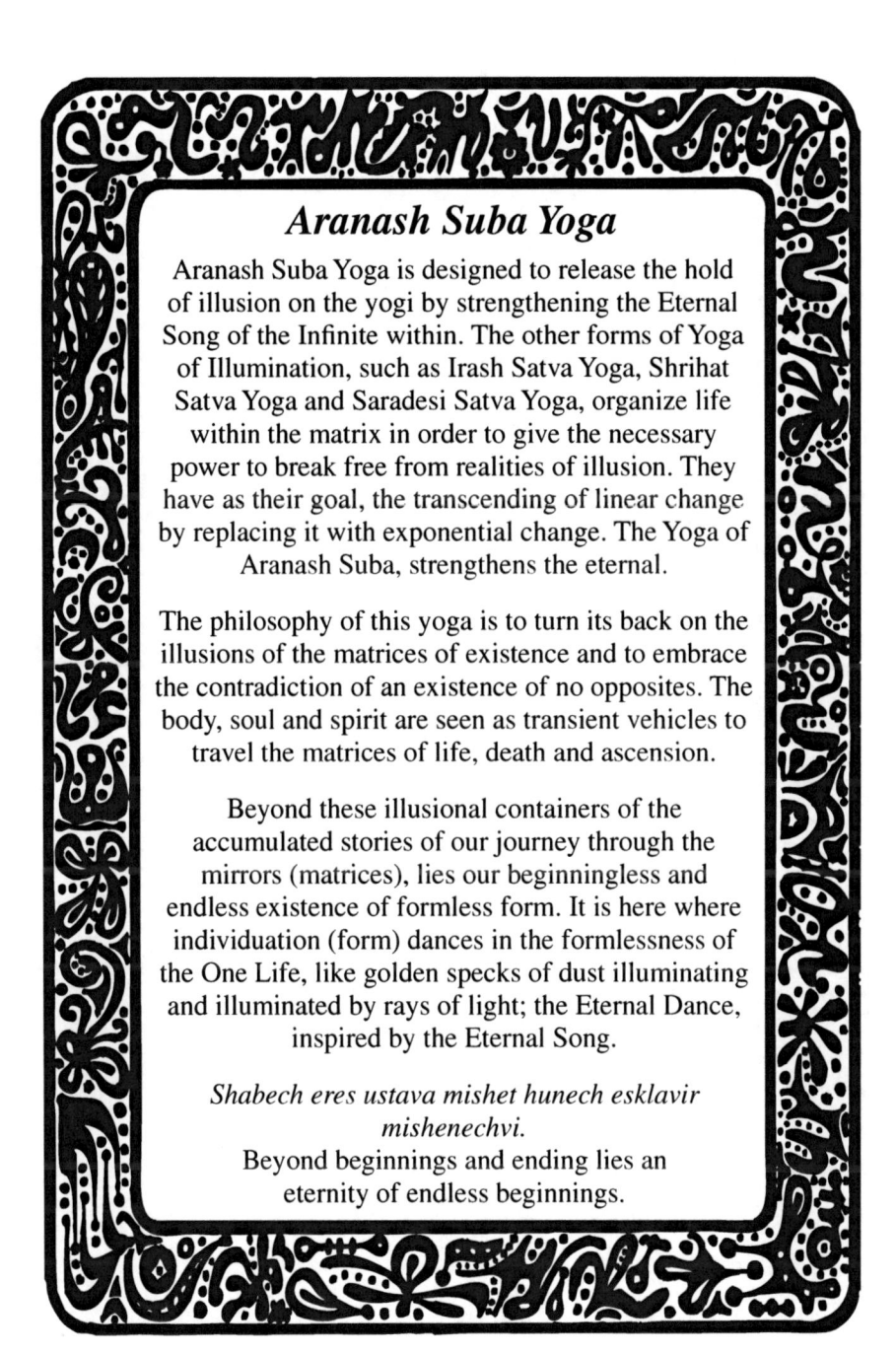

## *Aranash Suba Yoga*

Aranash Suba Yoga is designed to release the hold of illusion on the yogi by strengthening the Eternal Song of the Infinite within. The other forms of Yoga of Illumination, such as Irash Satva Yoga, Shrihat Satva Yoga and Saradesi Satva Yoga, organize life within the matrix in order to give the necessary power to break free from realities of illusion. They have as their goal, the transcending of linear change by replacing it with exponential change. The Yoga of Aranash Suba, strengthens the eternal.

The philosophy of this yoga is to turn its back on the illusions of the matrices of existence and to embrace the contradiction of an existence of no opposites. The body, soul and spirit are seen as transient vehicles to travel the matrices of life, death and ascension.

Beyond these illusional containers of the accumulated stories of our journey through the mirrors (matrices), lies our beginningless and endless existence of formless form. It is here where individuation (form) dances in the formlessness of the One Life, like golden specks of dust illuminating and illuminated by rays of light; the Eternal Dance, inspired by the Eternal Song.

*Shabech eres ustava mishet hunech esklavir mishenechvi.*
Beyond beginnings and ending lies an eternity of endless beginnings.

# How to do the Yoga

- Yoga mats are helpful for most of the yoga postures with the exception of posture 8 which requires a sturdy wall space for each participant to lean against.
- The first position of each set of postures (except postures 9 and 10) is accompanied by a meditation.
- The meditation postures: Hold the posture while contemplating the concept given. The concepts are specifically synchronized with the parts of the body that you will be stretching and are designed to release the tension of linear time and the resistance to life that are held there.
- The stretch postures: During the stretches you are no longer contemplating the associated concept used during the meditation posture. Feel the muscles and joints respond to the stretch with complete awareness while remaining fully present to the experience.
- The psoas muscle: This muscle holds the traumas of birth, death and the stages of ascension. The release of these traumas may be felt as involuntary muscle contractions and can occur during or even after the last few yoga positions are complete. Each person's response to the release of trauma held in the psoas muscle is unique; therefore you may want to allow an additional ½ hour lying down following the end of the session. This is especially true after the first session.
- The music/ yoga sound elixirs: The sound elixirs to be used with this yoga are balanced in black and white sound, which means that it assists in the release of past trauma and other illusions. It is the only music to be used with the yoga; bells indicate when to

change from one position to the next, from the meditation to the stretch postures as appropriate.
- When doing yoga it is important to respect your body. Only do what is comfortable for you, especially if you have not done yoga before. Do not force the postures nor hold them for longer than is comfortable. If you need to, return to a resting position and resume the posture when you feel you can. Over time you will be able to hold the posture for the full time.

# General Guidelines for Yoga

Wear comfortable clothing to allow for unrestricted movement.

Warm up muscles as you would for any exercise, with a few simple stretches to avoid injury or strain.

Ensure the environment is warm and comfortable.

Ease into postures and stretches with slow steady movements to the point of maximum effort. Listen to your body,

Breathing: Mindful breathing assists with relaxation of the body and maximum benefits with yoga. Breathe slowly and steadily, in through your nose and out through your mouth throughout.

A small pillow, folded towel and/or blanket may be useful for sitting postures and for the relaxation period at the end of the yoga session.

## The Psoas Muscle

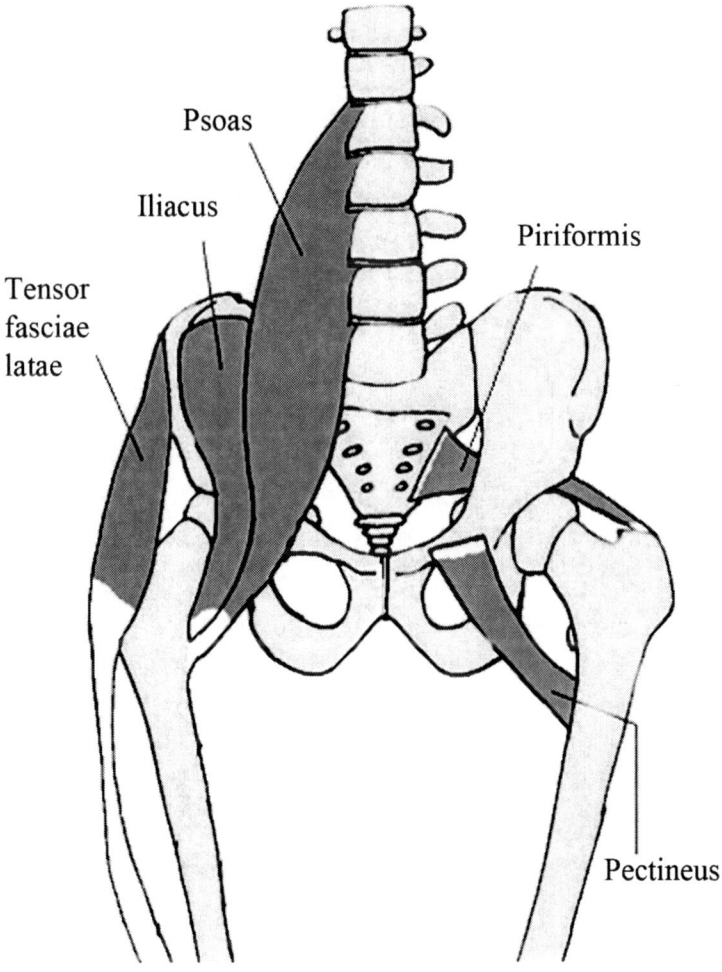

# Becoming the Contradiction
## Answers without Questions

This yoga is designed to create freedom from the tyranny of the matrices of human boundaries. It reaches where mind cannot go. The yoga practitioner learns to dance with the contradiction of the unanswerable, until eventually he steps off the treadmill of duality.

Initially, the contradiction and all its unanswerable nuances are pondered. Then, he or she dances with the contradiction by examining the question from all possible angles without deducing any meaning, nor arriving at any conclusion. It is simply observed that multiple answers exist, depending on what level the question is examined from.

Eventually, the practitioner becomes the contradiction by approaching it from deep core awareness and meditation, until the question itself disappears in the face of an unformulated knowing.

It is recommended that one of these proposed contradictory questions or answers be meditated on prior to doing the yoga. It is briefly observed with awareness after the yoga practice. This allows the practitioner to realize that with deep awareness beyond the question, subtle shifts can be felt.

*Anything that can be explained, is an imagined fabrication of the mind. The timeless, and inseparable, must be felt.*

# Dancing with the Contradiction

*Shebech mishanach ushech paru mesetet iklesh bravabruch?*
*Shebevech nuchsava pihavech kilshavechna truhabat.*

How can the eternal have more value than the transient when there is no time?
Anything that has an opposite is a fabrication of the mind.

*Menut hasbaaa eshevich stabahus?*
*Stravich meshech nasat stuhut ubavechvi.*

Am I walking across the ground?
Perhaps the earth moves beneath me from my intent.

*Shebech bruhu aras pravi mesenech stahurusatvi?*
*Shebehech setrech manitvi eruash sparuk eseklet.*

How can my choices affect all life when I have no freedom of choice?
All dwells within me and I dwell within all.

*Shperuch kyaket neneshut brisparek eklet hartu subavat?*
*Mechba bruhata setre irklavet hustechbi.*

If words are the veils that hide eternity, do they also frame it?
The Infinite can be seen only when viewed through the web of the finite.

*Sheberach nansat vartu blihas uspekve birestrechvi?*
*Ki harustach nenset parush misekletvi aruras paranut hursta.*

What is eternity, but a moment without boundary?
Nothing can be measured within the boundlessness of true existence.

PART I

# The Yoga Postures

# *Aranash Suba Yoga*

## *The Yoga of Enlightenment*

The first position of each posture set is to be held while meditating on the relevant concepts. Do not meditate while doing the stretches; be present to the experience. The audio recording that accompanies this yoga is the only music to be used; bells indicate when to change from one position to the next, from the meditation to the stretch postures as appropriate. The positions of each posture set 1 – 8 is held for 3 minutes. Postures 9 and 10 are held for 6 minutes each.

*The Yoga Postures*

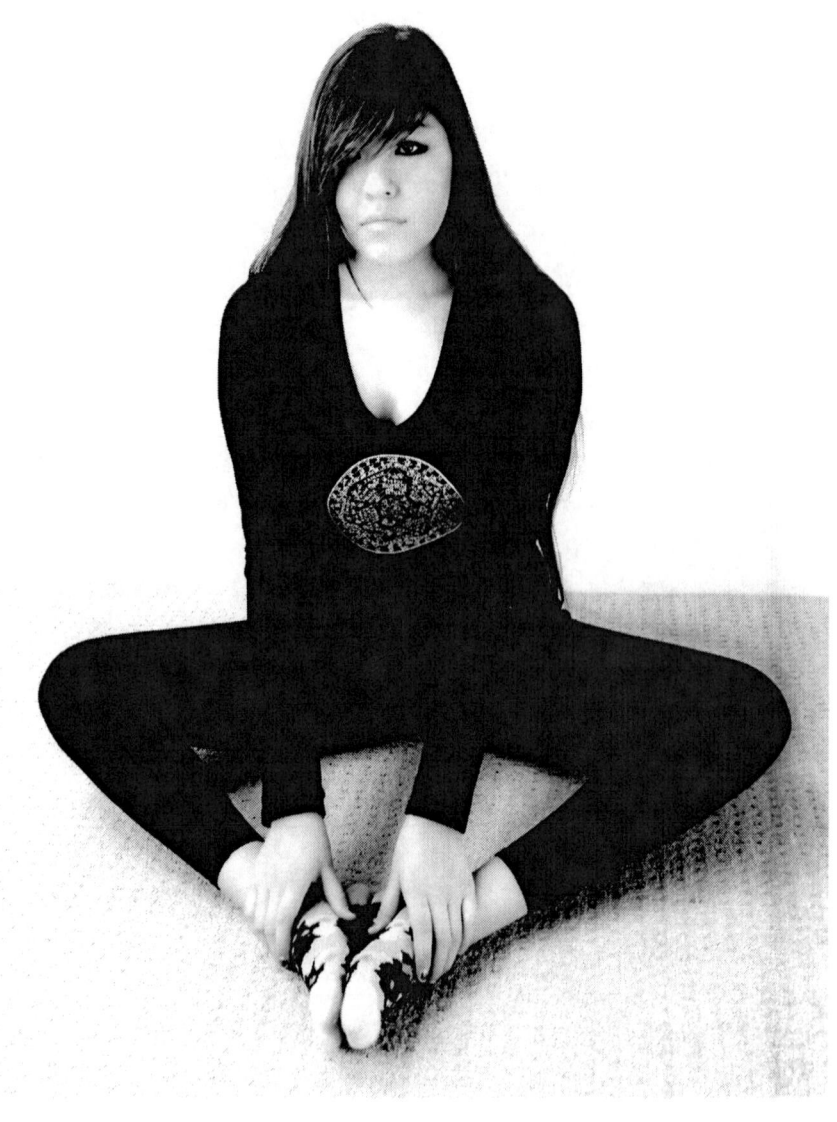

# 1. Posture name: Mechba-surat

## Posture – hold for 3 minutes
- Sit on the floor with your spine straight and your head facing straight forward.
- Bend your knees and bring the bottoms of your feet together with your knees out to the side.
- Rest your hands loosely on top of your feet with your palms down.

## Meditate on the following concept:
In guiltless perfection, existence unfolds. There is no good and evil beyond the matrices created by our belief systems. Individuations dance like flecks of dust in a light beam that shines through a window. The window consists of the mirrors of body, soul and spirit. In examining Itself, the Infinite cannot perceive Itself directly, the way a light beam cannot be seen directly. Only in observing the individuations that are illuminated by the light, can It be traced. Like dust in a light beam, there is no guilt or culpability – just aspects of life that from our vantage point, are incomprehensible.

## The Yoga Postures

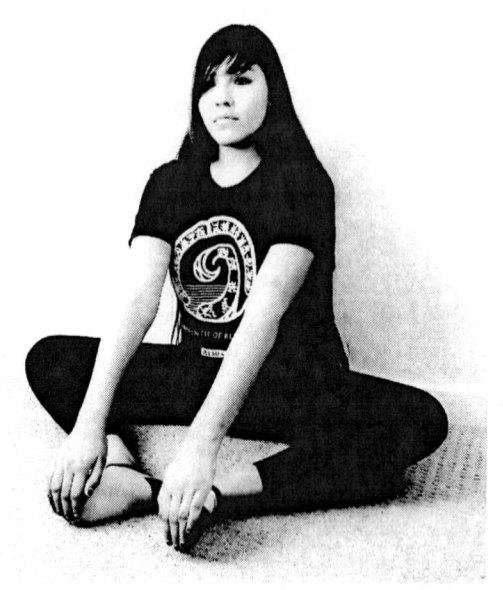

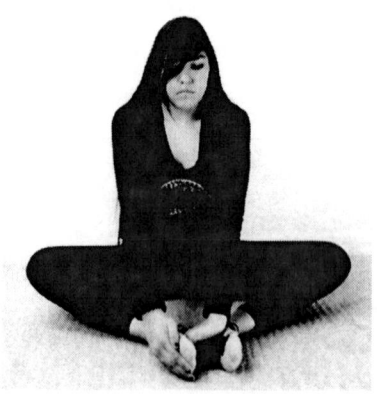
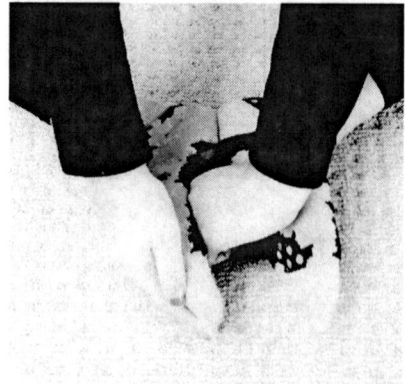

## Stretch for Posture 1 – duration 3 minutes

Maintain the same posture, alternate the following stretches of the feet, holding each stretch for a count of 20 seconds:

- Stretch 1. Keeping your heels together, grasp the balls of your feet with your hands and lift them upwards and outwards, away from each other. Keeping the heels together and maintaining the v-shape, creates flexion at the ankles. The toes are bent upwards by the pressure of your hands. Hold for 20 seconds.
- Stretch 2. Start with your left foot: while keeping your heels together and your feet in the v-shape, press your right fist in the ball of your foot. As you push your foot outwards with your fist, use your other hand to press the top of your foot and toes inwards, creating a stretch in your foot. Hold the stretch for 20 seconds.
- Stretch 3. Then repeat stretch 2 on the other foot. Again hold for 20 seconds.

Alternate these three stretches in sequence three times. Then rest with the bottoms of your feet together, in the original posture, for the remainder of the track

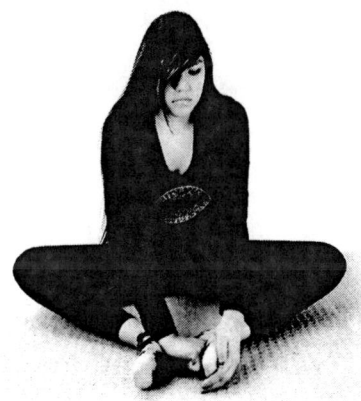
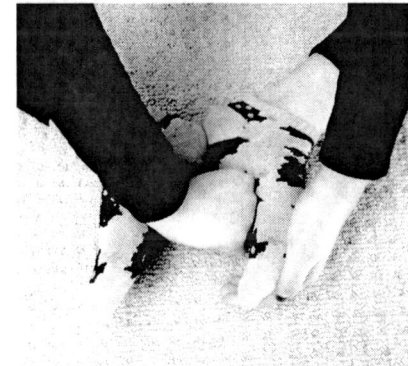

*The Yoga Postures*

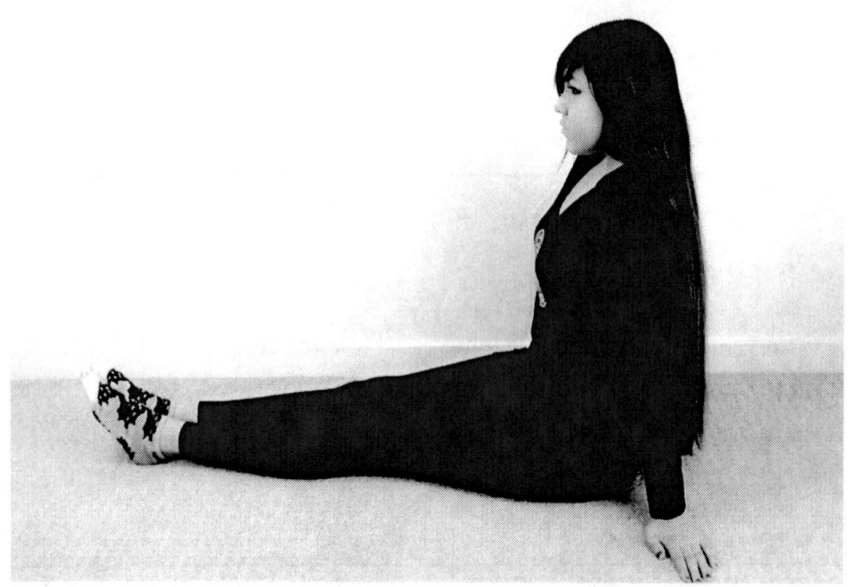

## 2. Posture name: Hirat-suvavi

## Posture – hold for 3 minutes
- In a seated posture with your spine and head straight, extend your legs straight out in front of you, keeping them together. Your feet will be in a relaxed position.
- Place your arms by your sides, palms on the floor.

## Meditate on the following concept:
It is the privilege of each being to illuminate the Infinite's ray of light with the dance of his or her existence. There is only the choice of dancing with grace through complete surrender, or of bouncing off the window of the mirrored matrices through opposing life. Let go the burdens of having to prove yourself, or fix or save others. Let your accomplishments be for the joy and adventure of life, all the while remembering that there is only the endless dance of eternal existence.

*The Yoga Postures*

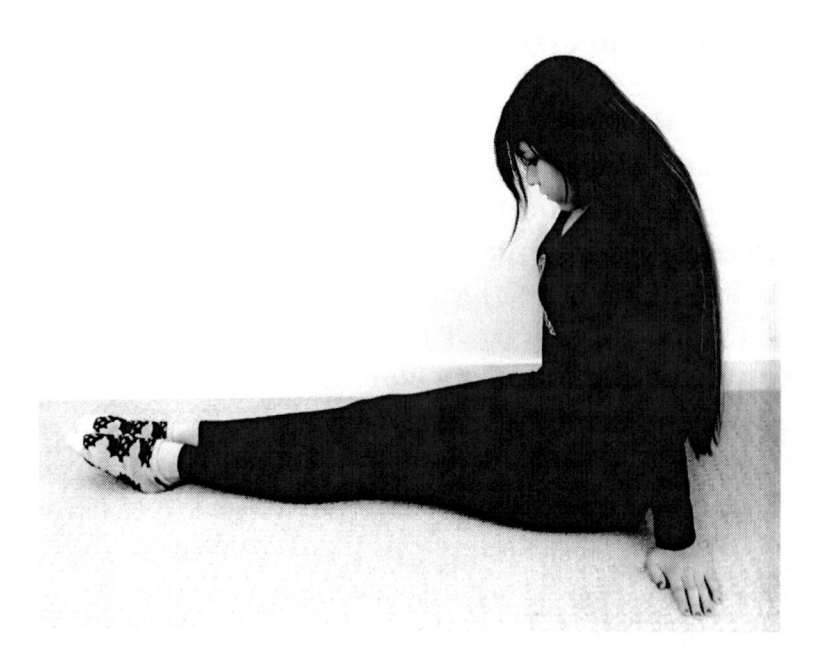

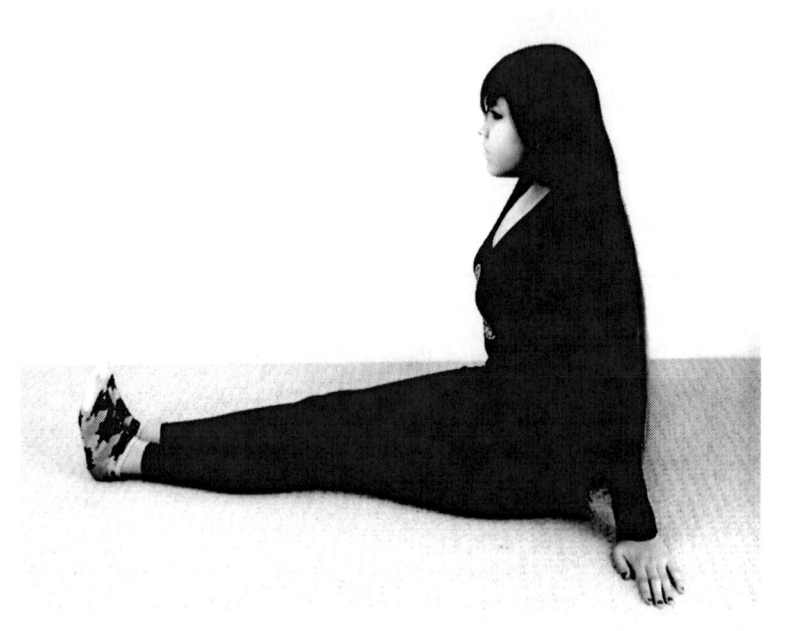

## Stretch for Posture 2 – duration 3 minutes
- Stretch 1. Sit on the floor with legs extended straight out in front of you with your feet together, toes pointing downward towards the ground as far as possible. Drop your chin onto your chest. Hold this stretch for 20 seconds.
- Stretch 2. Flex your ankles, pointing your toes towards your head as far as possible, creating a strong pull in your calves. Raise your head so your chin is level to the floor. Hold for 20 seconds.

Alternate these two stretches, all the while bracing yourself with your arms.

*The Yoga Postures*

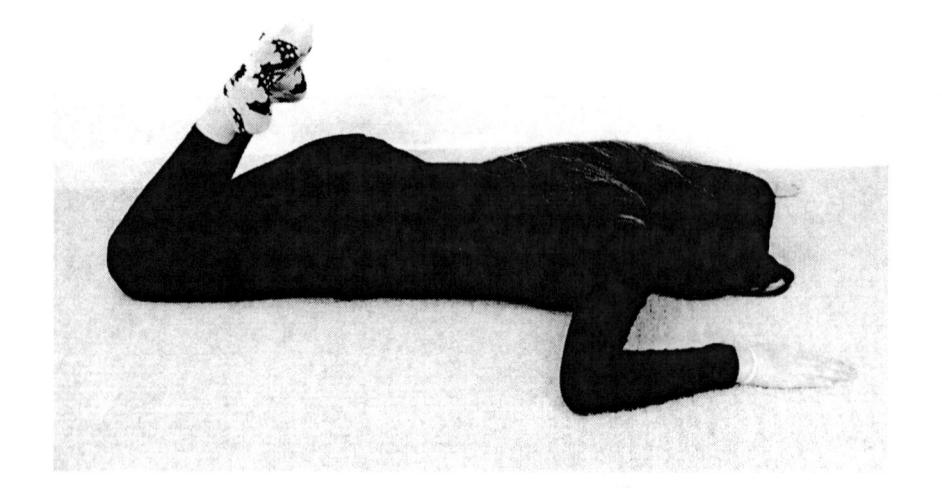

## 3. Posture name: Baruk-hespata

## Posture – hold for 3 minutes
- Lie on your stomach with your knees bent and shoulder-width apart.
- Point your toes as far as you can towards your head.
- Elbows are bent with your hands resting (palms down) on the floor next to your ears, approxiamtely shoulder-width apart.
- Your forehead rests on the ground.

## Meditate on the following concept:
Release now the addiction to form and let go of the tension that sustains it. The vehicles of body, soul and spirit are transient. Beyond these tools of expression, exists the realness of your being that has had neither beginning nor end. Embrace the timelessness of your infinite existence and the harmlessness of life shall reveal itself to you.

*The Yoga Postures*

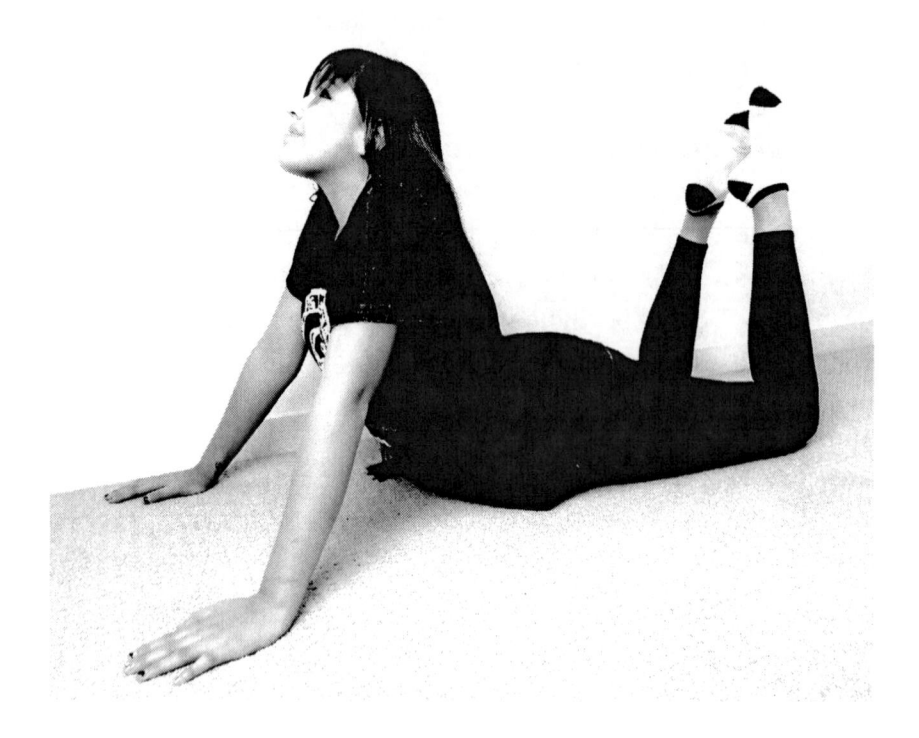

## Stretch for Posture 3 – duration 3 minutes

- Using your hands, push your upper torso up off the ground and bend your head back towards your feet. Your pelvis remains on the ground.
- Keep you feet pointed towards your head.
- You must feel a strong stretch in the front of your thighs.
- Hold this stretch for 20 seconds and then lower your upper torso back to the floor.
- Repeat the stretch 3 times, holding it for 20 seconds each time.

*The Yoga Postures*

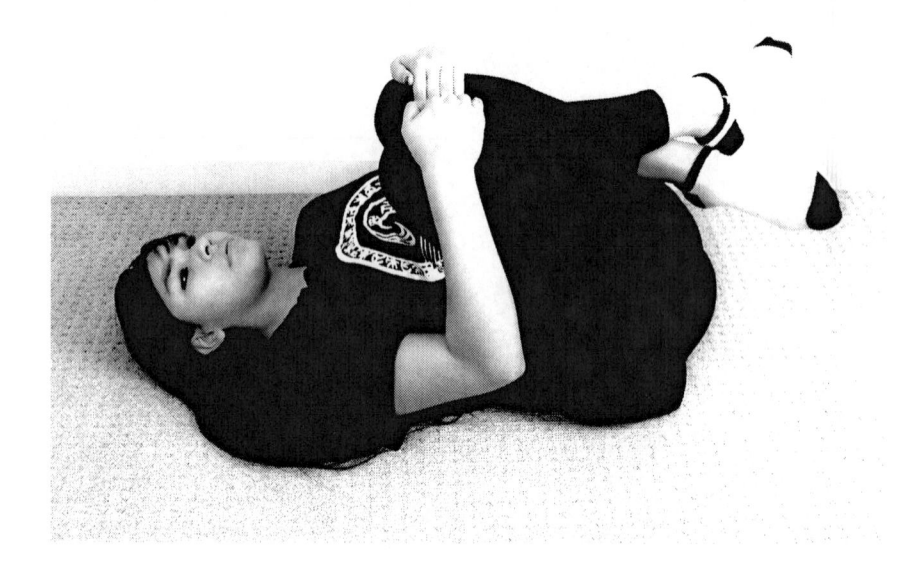

## 4. Posture Name: Spabak-miravetvi

### Posture – hold for 3 minutes
- Lie flat on your back with your knees bent and shoulder-width apart.
- Draw your knees up towards your chest (keeping them shoulder-width apart) and cross your ankles, placing whichever foot on top that is most comfortable.
- Grasp your shins by wrapping your arms around the outside of your legs.

### Meditate on the following concept
See yourself no longer as a body, a soul or a spirit, but rather as a timeless moving field of luminosity. Golden specks dance within your being – these too you are. All individuals dwell within the vastness of your being. Yet the true core of all individuals you are also.

*The Yoga Postures*

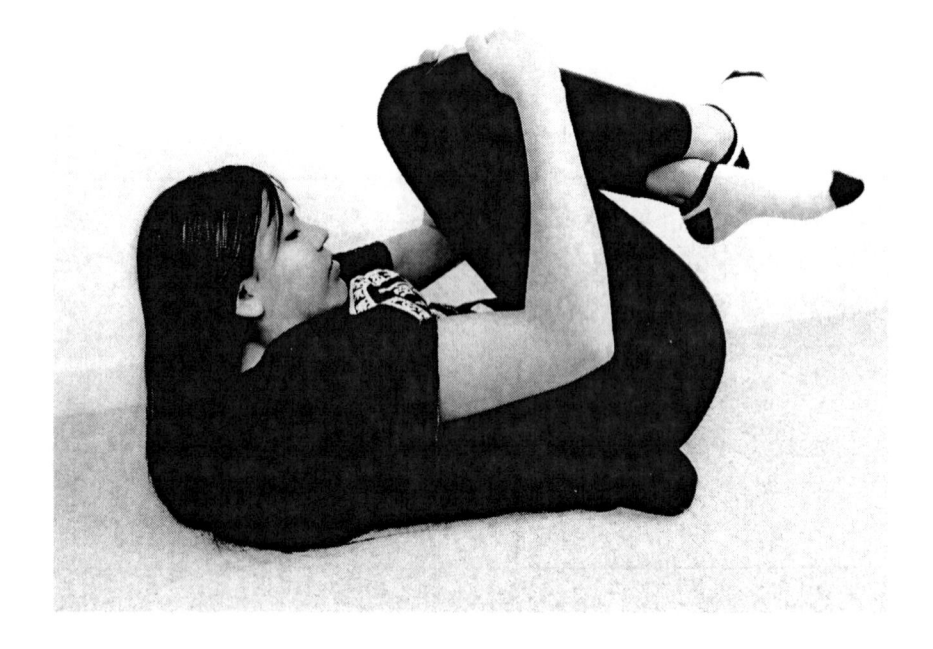

## Stretch for Posture 4 – duration 3 minutes
- Pull your knees towards your chest as hard as you can and curl your back and head up slightly. Sustain this posture for 20 seconds.
- Release your back onto the floor while continuing to pull your knees towards your chest with your hands and keeping your ankles crossed. Relax your back and neck as you lower your head to the floor, but continue to feel the pull in your buttocks. Sustain this posture for 20 seconds.
- Repeat both postures alternating between them.

*The Yoga Postures*

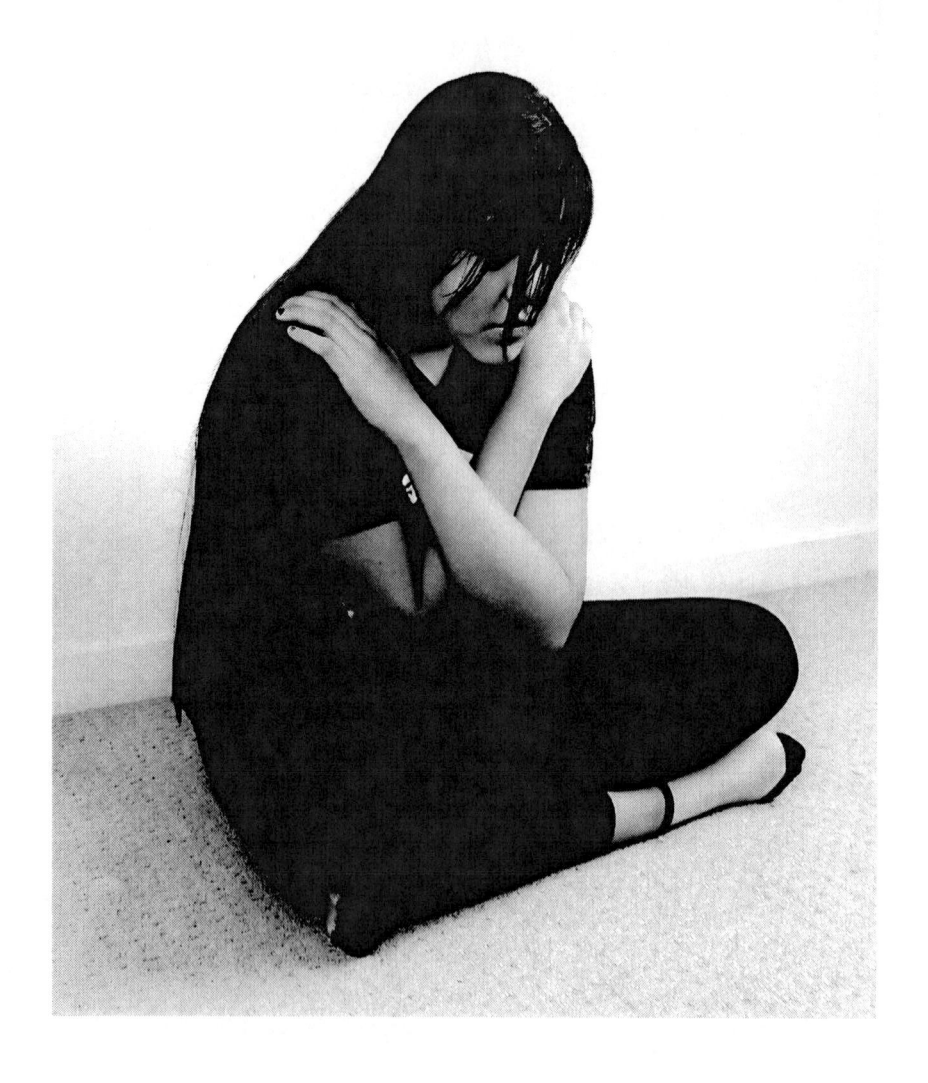

## 5. Posture Name: Krenit-usava

## Posture – hold for 3 minutes
- Sit on the floor in a comfortable position with your spine straight and your legs crossed. As you drop you legs out to the side, feel a slight stretch in your upper thighs and lower back (hint – move your feet toward the body to feel this stretch).
- Grasp your right shoulder with your left hand and the left shoulder with your right hand (use whichever arm is the most comfortable to have on the outside) and lower your chin to your chest.

## Meditate on the following concept:
Release the stories of your life and the need to be identified by what you do, what you have done, or personality traits. The personality traits are simply the coping mechanisms you have developed over ages of going around and around the matrix. See yourself as being genderless, identityless, and timeless. Release sentimental attachments; for it is only in releasing the emotional attachments to that which you hold most dear, that you will evolve beyond duality. All life shall be blessed when you do.

*The Yoga Postures*

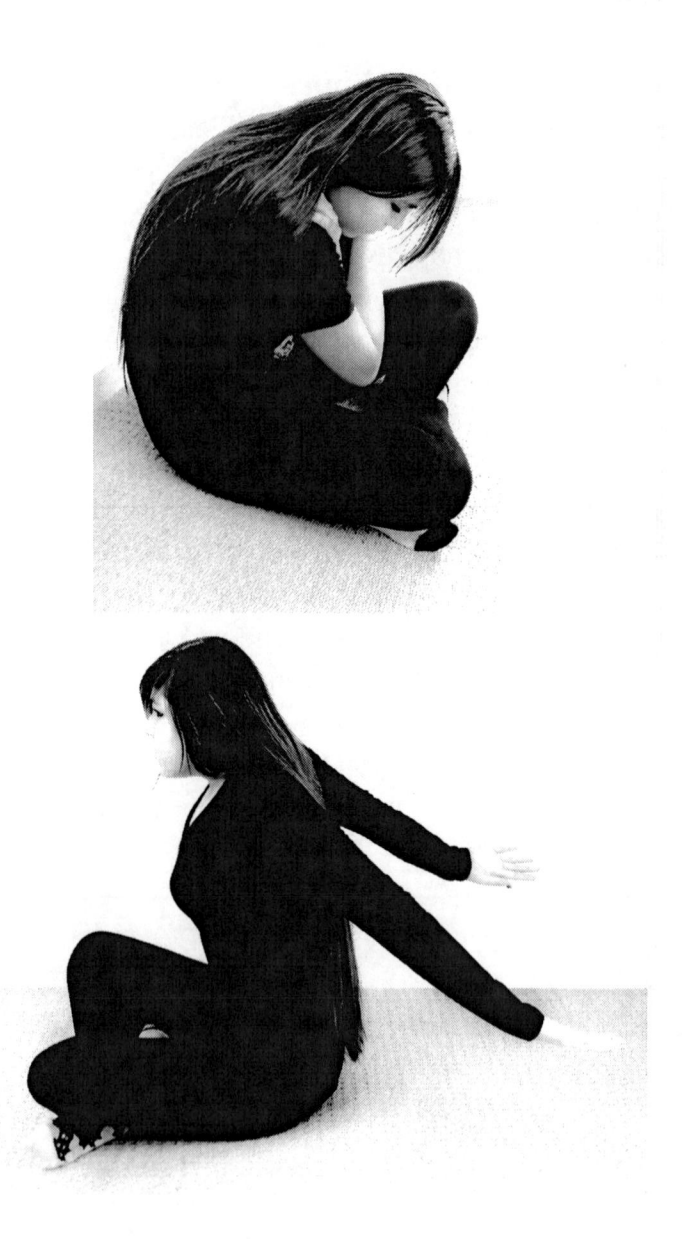

## Stretch for Posture 5 – duration 3 minutes
- Stretch 1. Staying in the same position, with your head on your chest and your arms grasping the opposite shoulder, arch (round) your back as far as you can. Keep your buttocks on the floor and your legs crossed in a comfortable stretch. Hold the arched back in a sustained position for 20 seconds.
- Stretch 2. Straighten your back and lift your chin, holding your head level. Keeping your arms straight and your palms facing upwards, bring your arms behind your back as far as they will go. Your hands should be shoulder-width apart. Feel the stretch in your chest. Hold this posture for 20 seconds.
- Return to the original posture of arching your back and grasping the opposite shoulders. Remember to lower your chin onto your chest. Hold this posture again for 20 seconds
- Alternate between these two postures for the duration of the track.

*The Yoga Postures*

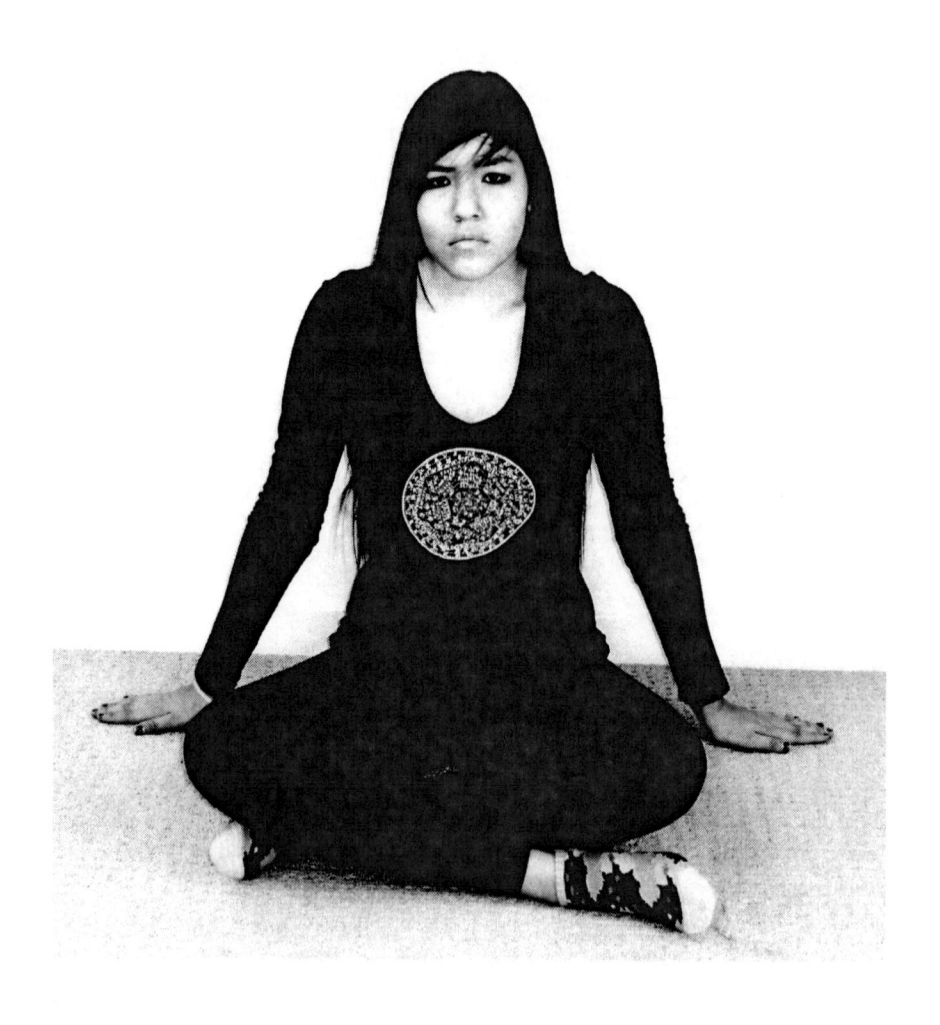

## 6. Posture Name: Meshak-blavablut

## Posture – hold for 3 minutes
- Sitting with your legs crossed in a comfortable stretch and your spine straight, move your arms out by your sides. Rest them gently on the floor (palms down) with your elbows straight. Keep you chin up and your head level.

## Meditate on the following concept:
You are the center of your reality. All you can ever know is your reality. Allow yourself to know that as anything changes within, so everything in your reality has to change likewise. Compare it to a tube full of marbles. If you add one more marble in one end, no matter how long the tube is, all marbles must shift, dropping one out at the opposite end. Know yourself not only as the center of your reality but as a grounding rod for all life within it. The pranic tube extends from your crown through the base of your spine. It is that which grounds the electrical energy of the activity of the world around you, as well as the magnetic energy of all the seething emotions of humanity and beyond. As a grounding rod, you prevent catastrophes as a method of bringing forced change. As long as you live from the center of your reality, as the grounding rod of all life within it, catastrophic events are averted.

*The Yoga Postures*

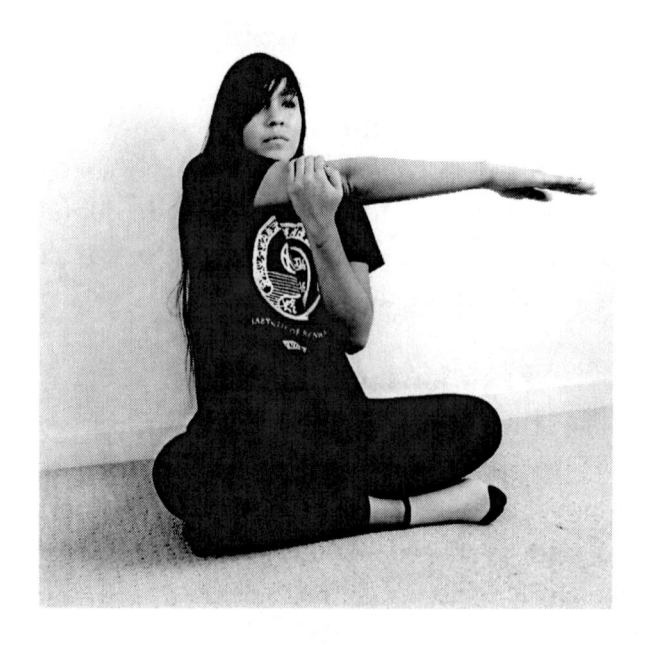

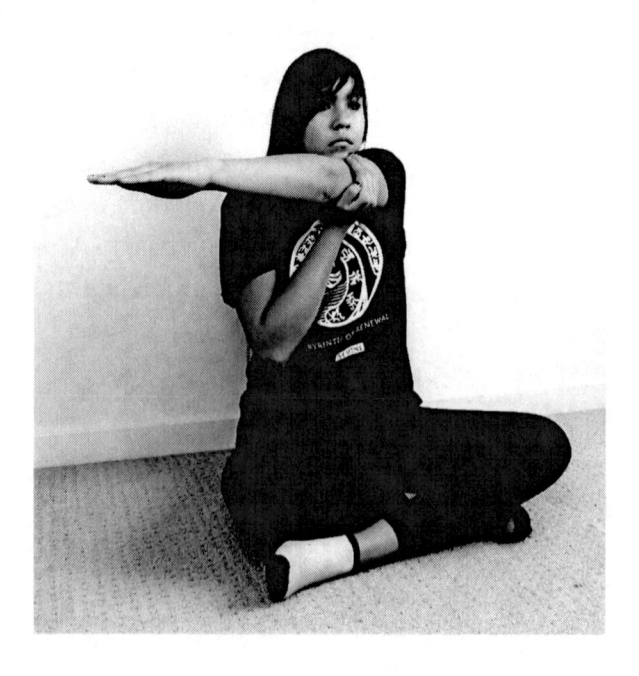

## Stretch for Posture 6 – duration 3 minutes
- Extend your straightened right arm across your chest to the left. With your left hand, press on your upper arm from underneath to increase the stretch. Hold this for 20 seconds.
- Now repeat the exact same stretch on the opposite side by pushing against your extended left arm. Hold for 20 seconds.
- Repeat these stretches by alternating between your right arm and your left arm for the duration of the elixir.

*The Yoga Postures*

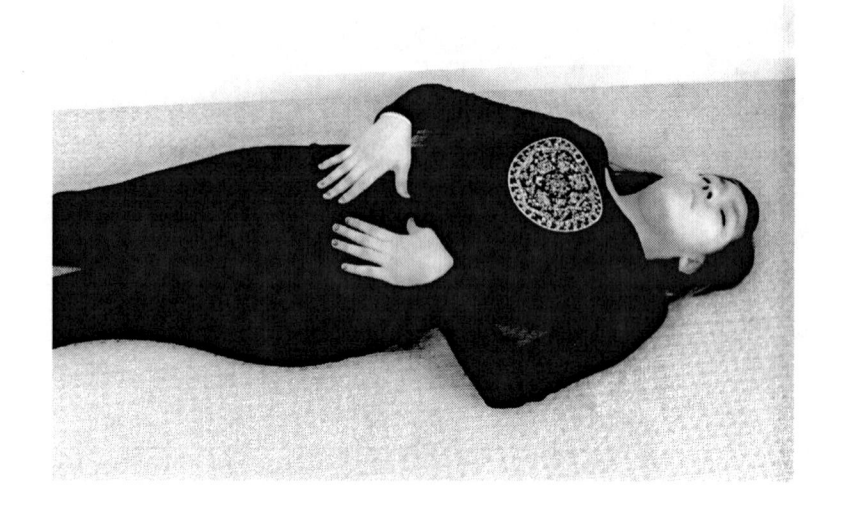

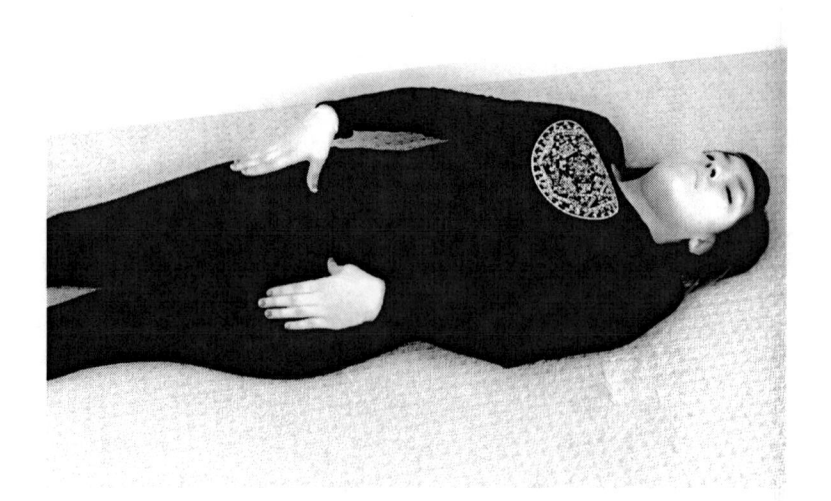

# 7. Posture Name: Brishbaranut-usaba

## Posture – duration 3 minutes
- Lie flat on your back with your legs straight out in front of you and your feet approximately 6 inches apart.
- Place your thumbs on your waistline, approximately 1 inch from your navel on either side. Your right thumb will be 1 inch to the right of your naval and your left thumb will be 1 inch to the left.
- Push on these points with your thumbs. As you contemplate the meditation, slowly move your thumbs outwards in a V-pattern, 45 degrees down and out towards your hips until level with the pubic bone.
- Repeat this same movement from either side of your navel down towards your hips over and over again with very slow movements for the duration of the elixir.

## Meditate on the following concepts:
Imagine yourself as an ocean of luminosity, as vast as existence. See yourself turn your attention to various locations within your vastness. As there is slight intention directed at a specific part of the ocean, it lights up even more. Maintain the concept of having no boundaries as you notice that, like the ocean, there is no linear movement – just formlessness forming in ever-changing ways. Although the shoreless ocean of your being has no boundaries and there is no directionality in its movements, yet it appears to be ever moving although it is traveling nowhere. Envision this within the vastness of your own being.

*The Yoga Postures*

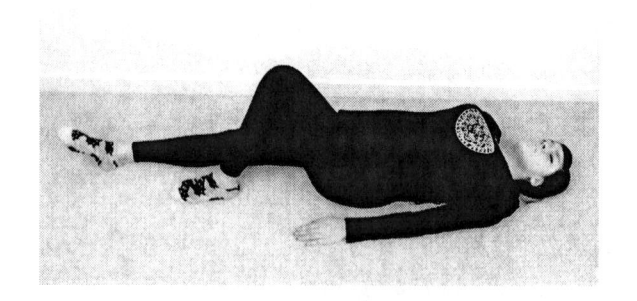

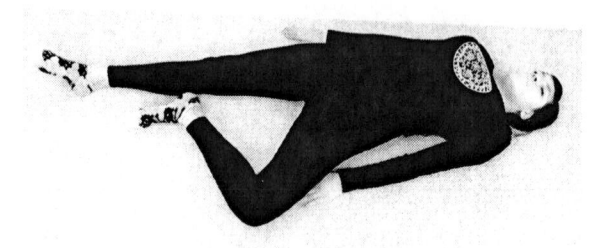

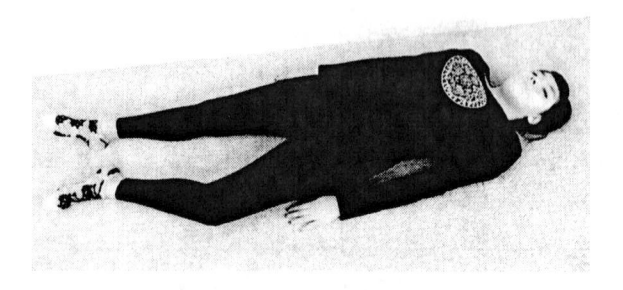

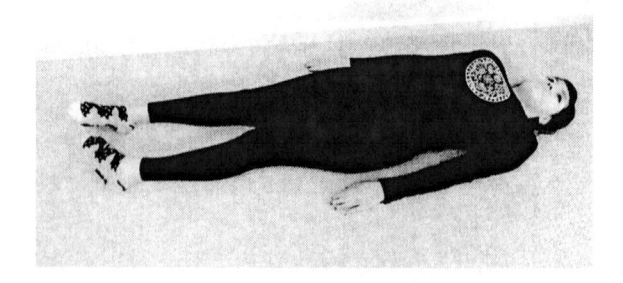

## Stretch for Posture 7 – duration 3 minutes
**Note:** If you have any discomfort in one of your hips, sciatica on one side, or a pain in one of the buttock muscles, begin the stretch with the opposite leg to the one that has the discomfort.

- Bring your leg upwards until your knee is bent and pointed towards the ceiling. The other leg remains flat and relaxed upon the ground.
- When your knee is bent to its maximum capacity, drop your leg out to the side as far as it will go. The right leg will move towards the right side, or the left leg to the left side, depending on which leg you chose to start with.
- When you have extended your bent leg as far towards the side as provides a comfortable stretch, straighten the leg out while keeping the knee facing toward the side, until it is completely straight. Your foot should be 6 inches away from your other leg.
- Then, flip the ankle of the leg you are working with, inward so that your toes are pointed in towards the opposite foot. Hold this for 10 seconds.
- Repeat the same procedure with the other leg.
- Repeat this stretch, alternating between your right and left leg, for the remainder of track.

*The Yoga Postures*

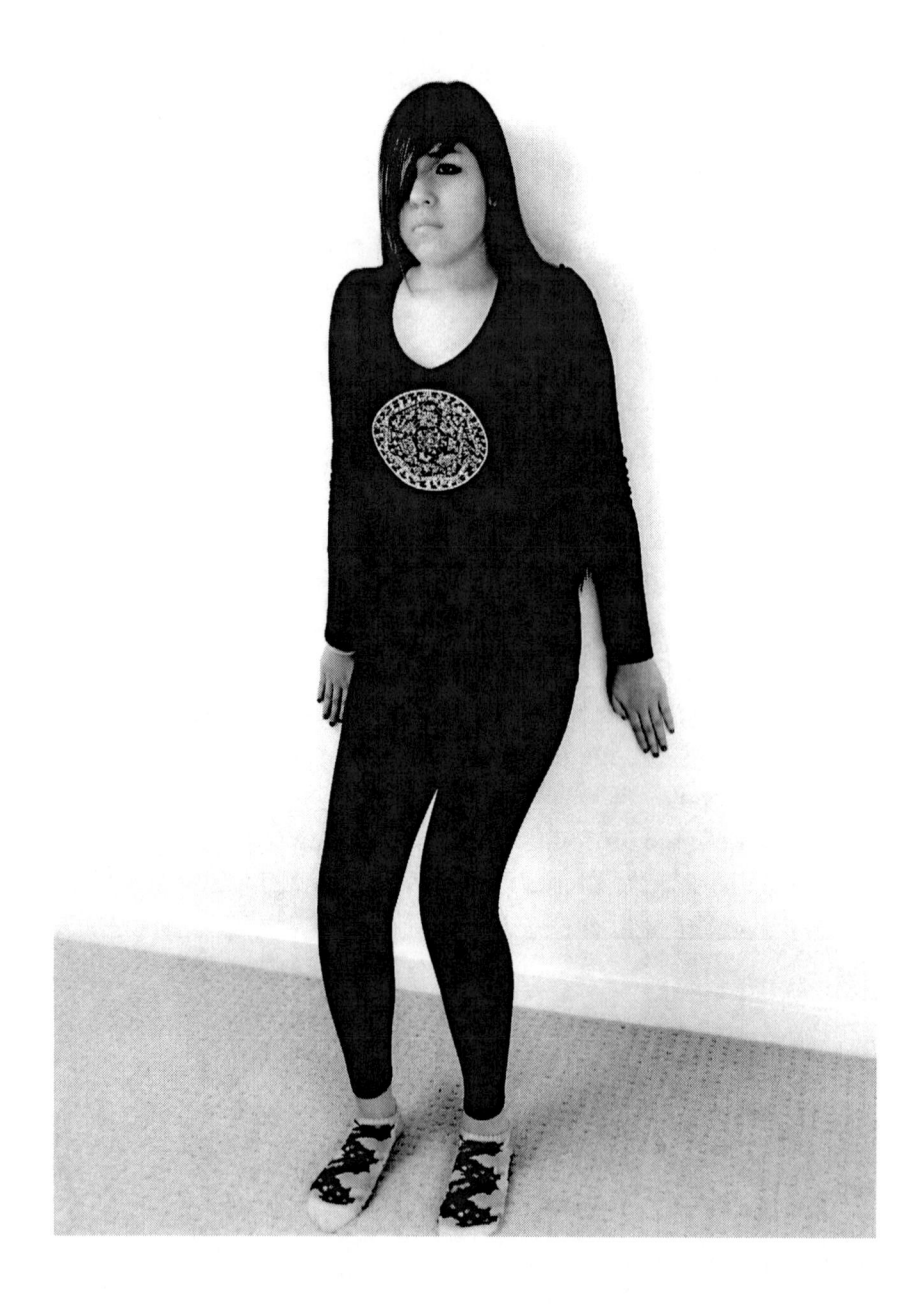

# 8. Posture Name: Machtu-nenesh-bravut

## Posture – hold for 3 minutes

Stand with your back (entire spine) against a wall with your knees slightly bent and your palms against the wall, feet slightly out from the wall. Your arms will be straight and your chin level with the ground.

## Meditate on the following concepts:

Imagine yourself as a specific current that fills the boundless ocean of the One Life. Feel the subtle shifts within eternity. Great changes happen on the surface (your every day life) as the subtle currents flow at the deepest level of the ocean. As you feel these subtle shifts, know that they are creating new expressions every second on the surface appearances of existence.

*The Yoga Postures*

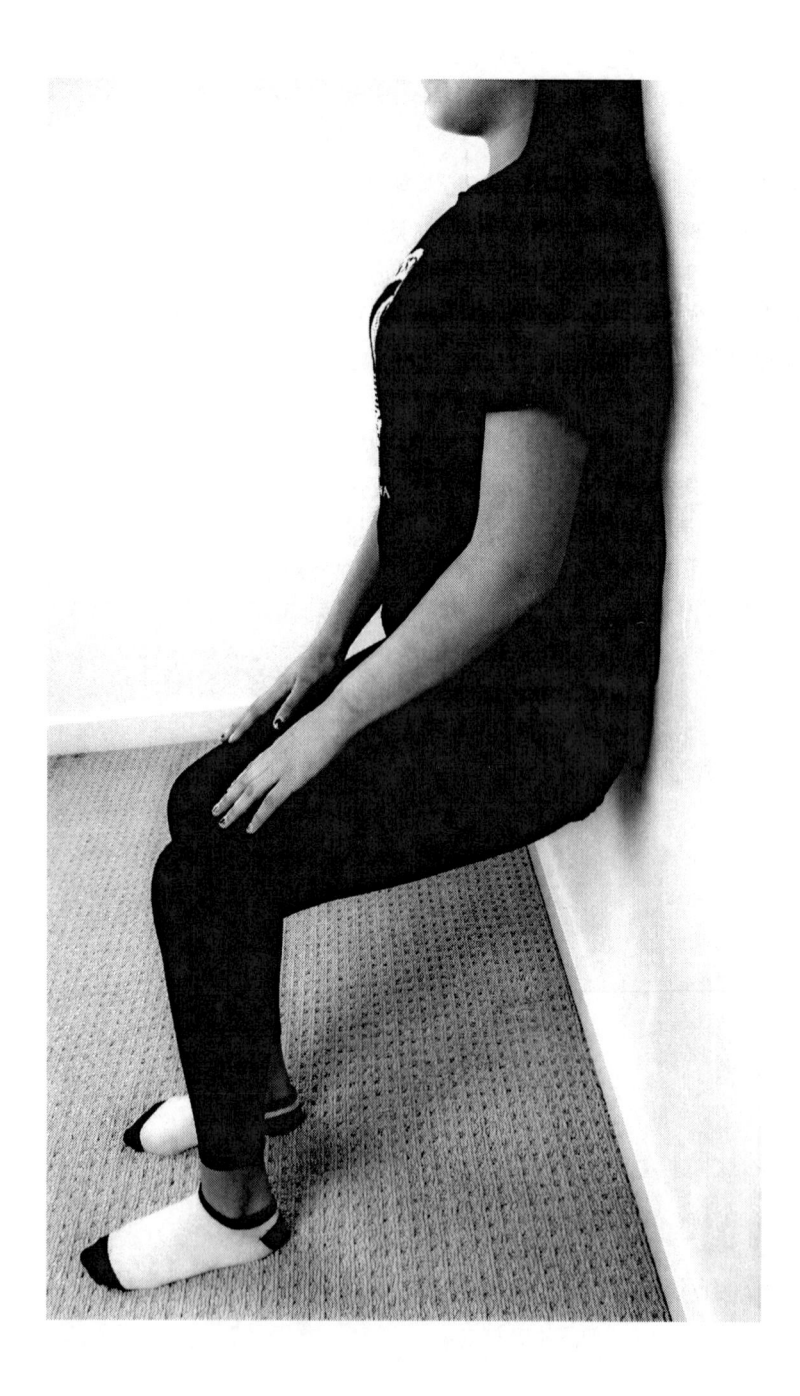

## Stretch for Posture 8 – hold for 3 minutes
- Place your hands lightly on your knees and move your feet out in front of you. With your back pressing firmly against the wall, slide down the wall gradually as far as you can while still <u>comfortably</u> supporting yourself. Ensure that your knees are in line with your feet; your feet should always be in front of the knees to avoid knee strain.
- Only do what is comfortable for you. If you find the stretch difficult, return to a standing position and when your body has relaxed, return to the stretch again.
- The aim is to maintain a stretch where you appear to be sitting on an invisible chair, with you thighs parallel to the floor and your knees at a 90-degree angle.
- Hold this stretch for the duration of the track or as long as your feel is comfortable for you. Remember you may take a break in the middle and return to the stretch again.

*The Yoga Postures*

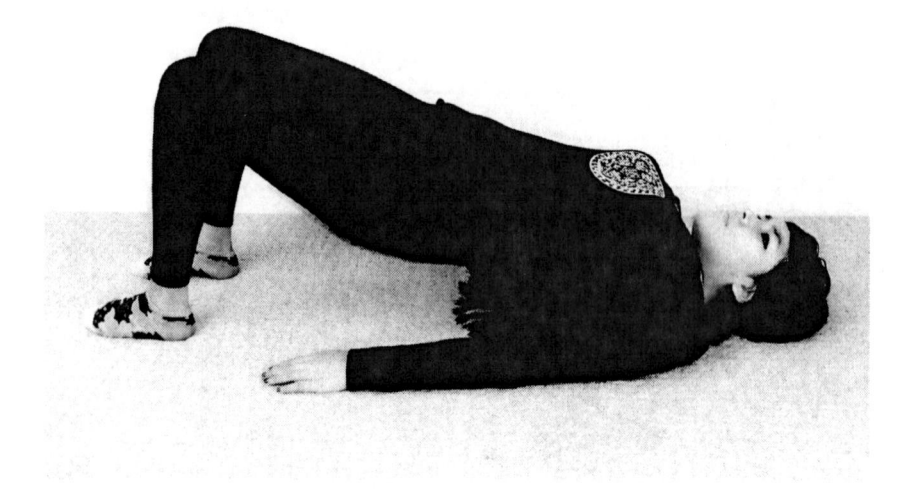

## 9. Posture Name: Plihasba-nanuk

## Posture – hold for 6 minutes
- Lie flat on your back, with your arms straight down by your side and your palms on the floor. Bend you knees and place your feet flat on the ground. Keep you feet shoulder-width apart.
- Raise your pelvis up from the ground as far as is comfortable for you.
- Hold this position for the duration of the track (6 minutes) or as long as you can comfortably do so. You may lower yourself onto the ground, have a rest and then return to the posture.

## Meditate on the following concepts:
Completely empty your mind and simply allow whatever involuntary movements your body chooses to make, to happen. If a thought arises, don't engage it. Simply observe it, the way a wave rises and falls on the crest of an ocean. Your body may at this point go into convulsive movements of the abdomen, experience contractions of the lower abdominal muscles or you may have the desire to rock back and forth.

**Note:** This posture is maintained for the duration of this part of the yoga. If no involuntary movements occur, do not feel that this posture has not been effective or that the yoga is not doing what it is designed to do. Yoga students vary widely in their response to this part of Aranash Suba Yoga. Lower your back to the floor, only if you can no longer support the raised pelvis. Try and keep it raised for the duration of this particular part of the yoga.

*The Yoga Postures*

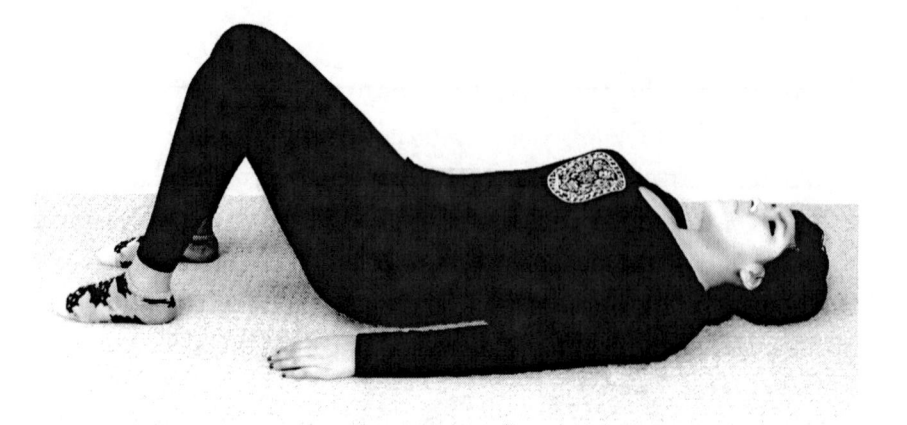

## 10. Posture Name: Bleshbit-urunachvi

## Posture – hold for 6 minutes

The posture for this final part of the yoga session is exactly the same as the previous one, except now you lower your back to the floor. Your back will be straight, and your arms will remain straight by your side. Your knees will be bent as they were in the previous position. Allow whatever involuntary movements may take place to occur, without trying to stifle or subdue them. Some yoga students have experienced convulsive type movements in the lower abdomen for up to an hour after the yoga has ended. If this is to occur, it is essential that you allow yourself time for this, until all movement has stopped.

Yoga students, who initially experience no involuntary movements, may experience them at a later date. This occurs because the yoga has removed layers of illusion and a new threshold has been reached. Know that whether the movements are experienced or not, the yoga will be equally effective in its results.

## Meditate on the following concept:

As with the previous posture, keep your mind as free from thought as possible. If a thought arises, don't engage it. Simply observe it, the way a wave rises and falls on the crest of an ocean.

PART II

# Related Insights from the Scrolls of Hanasat

# Insights into the Eternal Dance
# From the Scrolls of Hanasat

*Chirach mesete hunasvi sklarak*
*Prihesta vibrech suherestat unach*

Believe in nothing, for only then can you freely and effortlessly know.

∞

*Spiharach nesetu biresh privahet bires esekle huset. Virsabach uretvi karus pares minevesvi sekre utret paravi.*

Seek not meaning, for it retains that which has become meaningless. Perception without conclusion brings clarity.

*Brinavik usechvi mishet henasech brihet vibrech sparetvi nensarat husple ustavi vibrachvi*

As long as the judgment of good and bad exists, dictators will arise to defend or enforce their point of view.

*Mechpa nanuset herevesh arastu blivech sarsatu uhuvaset nusta habaset hurespi.*

Inspiration does not come in the form of an idea, but as a subtle, yet profound change in the song of your life.

*Shivahet ubrechvi minusat ekles harasparvi minech savatu shelehes vavit ekratbi minahes.*

Do not fear pain, for it is in pushing through and beyond it, that you will find greater joy.

∞

*Michta brisabek erekte-vi aras menetu plivechvi hersata minaves brivabek herestu anach selsava priviravech anesviva.*

Individuations are the seekers of self-beauty and wonderment within the eternal, undifferentiated flow of existence.

*Shebevich neskave prihat minasut blives estreve unas herspata vibrachvi sklerut aresta. Plihes nenes harspava vibrech sta-unit ereklesve virsh prahut nenechvi stahuvit aresta spivarech neneshtavu pli-es.*

Speak not to manipulate, control or persuade, but let your words be free from attached outcome. Your words are the veils that are drawn to reveal or conceal the never-ending mysteries of the Eternal Being.

∞

*Kirsava herestu minuvech vibrasvi ersaklut uras pirit uklet vibrasvi harsata ustech nunes blivabas arska. Krives nichvetur harsata mishenuch ubret prahasvi verenuch sahabit arevestu aranach.*

Taste becomes an addiction when it is used as a substitute to fill the gaps left by deprivation of touch. Explore your world with touch to receive its sacred alchemy of inspiration.

*Kersavach minusuch brivat herespi aklatva herestu minasuch vibresvi arasut. Nechspahur esekletvi mishtahur enestravi erech pahur nanunes.*

In speaking mind to mind, or even heart to heart, we speak the shallow words of deception. No two perspectives can converse, as the perspective of each is unique.

∞

*Nansklave misevech hunavesvi eruret blihavech eskre bravet sklava prihanes eresh asatu minevat skaravink.*

Let your words flow from the eternal silence of your infinite song, that the depth of your being may touch that of another between your words.

*Mesetu misanech herstu mishat arek navesbi plivahet eklestru mavech vilestra pravekvi eres nanustra. Kiva hes esetra mivavechspri arunas uvahespi.*

No separation can exist, therefore no relationship. The Infinite does not express or there would be a relationship between the expressed and the expresser. There is no such thing as creation; there is only the One Life.

∞

*Neksavu vibrechvi anas eres ukletvi berech baruk mishe netvi hersatu*

There is no meaning to primal existence, just the Eternal Self observing Itself.

*Sikrat nurnavi erekta plavabit arsanach set vileshva hurspahur nechta skrevileveshvi misenech setur na skri-uhurunat valeshvi uherevi. Nantach bires etrevanik beletre nanuchvra bilestur subatu mishenechvi.*

Eating is a sacred ritual that fulfills its holy purpose only in the silence of thoughtful contemplation, gratitude and sensitive awareness. The sense of taste inspires the notes of the Eternal Song.

∞

*Kelspahur sklehura nespava virsprechvu nanunish esekle prehut. Virsenech herus arsatva misech haruhet privavet vibech kranas suvit erekletvi minach hersetu vibret arunas klaharuvit vibret eres usta blivechvi verespa ste-unit.*

Touch is the way to explore life in a deeper manner. Allow yourself to feel with more than your skin. For in feeling an object, or another, with the fullness of your being, alchemy of inspired, exponential change occurs.

*Kelshavich visetret unas bliverevichva uhur nispavek vibrech stauharanit stelenechvi varsatur esenit kenuch virevespahur eselvi archpahur minavish hersetu skravele vispahur nuvataa uresvi.*

Be aware of what food you wish to reach for, since it serves the purpose, through taste, of inspiring into expression the full resonance of the indivisible and eternal that you are.

∞

*Kerenech suhatvi mishet anach suvetvi klihuset arava. Michtu vibrech eresvi ninusat kelesbi mistechvi hures aresta manusech blivabet areskva sihutvabi kri vanadech eresta hut mishet harestu eres harustach.*

The desire for tribalism, and the illusion of aloneness, keeps the imagined tribe of body, soul and spirit in place. The tribe promises support, but gives only as long as you permit them to control.

*Kruvavet suhetvi anas priheresta misenech kluvaset mihuranach. Krisepa stuvavi heretpavi ninusech paresta kiranet sevehut aresta misuhanech iklet vibret eret vanadoch.*

The core patterns of existence only flow when we cease anticipating possible outcomes. The large patterns of possible outcomes move into new probabilities when we respond day by day, from the silent strength of our indivisible being, to what is before us.

∞

*Nuchsabarek hestu erekla paruvit harchklava erus mananes huspava rukvetvi erestu manunech skrihu hersata mivet heres ustava vibrech sihuvavetvi miserech nastu. Stihublevesvi arkpa miserech nuset viranut. Plivech setrevu minash hersta huravet kla-unit brivahetspi erste nanutvi.*

The matrices of existence are still part of the Infinite Being's existence. The One Life expressing as the many, yet indivisible and eternal, is all there is. They are but temporary perspectives looking at specific aspects of Infinite Being.

*Pere-nuretvavi nuchte risetvi helshparanutvi ersekla bravahuravit estra miple krihu eresta kersvavi nech seleva heres vibrechta usit mishtavit erkletvi uvechvra-ur. Eretu plivaber nechtu surat privesbi ararat niserech.*

To create the perspectives, certain parts ceased participating in the unfolding self-revelation of the Infinite and became the observers. Their chance to participate has come.

∞

*Perehutva usach erenishtu hursat. Misenech hurpava eklet vibrestravu. Privebes erch klahunat visebrit menunech harsta arsanech hirstruvet. Siberutvi nenustat harsatu uret pretpravi arsanach.*

The non-participation of aspects of our eternal being arises when there are parts of ourselves we do not accept or value. We then live a programmed life.

*Verehuras asatra brihes uset pravech haravi mishevechvi nesatu uskle barut haresta pravadoch minaves heres eseklu prisenet elshklanut hares nesvavi ustechvi.*

The programs that we use to hide our 'unacceptable' expressions, become the identities we most vehemently defend. Self-love is the first step to identity-free mastery.

∞

*Kriharavit peleshestravi minach sivatur meshpavi ersetur hiravachvi blisbabek ekre suhat perevesvi unet. Santuvi-es kriharavishvi nanutach prihestravu skrihavet nanustar.*

The appreciative eyes of the master reveal the hallowed sacredness of life. The eyes of one who thinks he knows, affirm the shallow illusions of life.

*Selevish akratprahut sechva nestu haravis praheretat skrihauvi nenech suhar privesvi. Karchsavu minevit plihesvi araksta brivabech heres ursata viselenut selevishna-es.*

Sight is a doorway through which the real and eternal enters to perceive Itself. When sight believes it knows, it creates its own prison bars of belief systems.

∞

*Ursetpravahur nenek hiresta bravich eres kletvravir belestachvi nersba huretur pleva.*

When the real touches the real, rapture results and all of reality changes.

*Suvach heresat uras mishenat uhururespi skrihunat aklat vibres herenasvi krihunat sperech usetre vibresvi stra-unach subi.*

Until the fullness of expression can be reached, in which the input and output of your lives are inseparable, take time to experience both.

∞

*Krihanat uvaskelechna ubrechvi haranat kriharanas suvavi. Etre misanut krihastar eklech virsavat vibranes esekle hirset pri-avach nestasu krihuravespi estrehur arstanach misetvi.*

Man grieves that he gives much but does not receive much back. All the while he is closed to receiving because he does not allow himself the time to go into the depth of receptive silence.

*Chebehech setve anush usaba hanunik mivechva kerenut hanestra plivabich sevetvi urash. Nenseret plivech sahutbi iklet vinespahu.*

Food is used to fill the need for input when we do not allow it to occur through receptive silence. Because it is a substitute and cannot fulfill the need, it becomes an obsession.

∞

*Nersklerut erektrachvi virseblat minusech heres urstava blishet prehat areklatvi stra-uhes birseta. Rachnet bri-eklatur siberutpavi misenut havravesbi skelanot. Esklerut prehana sebevich estet manuvit.*

The four matrices of existence through which life rotates, and which in man forms the body, soul and spirit, were themselves formed when sight, hearing, feeling and touch separated from functioning as a whole. Smell never fell into separateness.

*Kreheshva achbravu unaves heras estavirechba hananus klivavesh hustra manunes urakspa vibrech stihubilesvit. Kersavi erek truhabis pliha vibrechspi anas hersatu minuhes uset minuvech.*

The re-establishing of vital and aware expression, of a more complete existence as a boundless being, has three steps. Realization of our previous reliance on illusion for guidance is the first step.

∞

*Prihat nenushta eksevat ekret prihatur husavesvi esklavach nisatve barasut husteva minech subahit eresach estubavi vileshvi. Hesklet uras visebretvi ekrech minuvit setlva misetut herenut eskravi.*

The creation of the perspectives (later becoming the body, soul and spirit) in order to observe an aspect of the eternal self's expression, became the dictators of how existence should unfold. All it could then behold was Itself and life became a mirror.

*Shehech navi seba ustava hereklesvi nanusit: Perek brava vires arsta nechvi suves uset varavi mineshvi skuhavat ereklash nanasut priherevas.*

The second step to evolve the interpretation of Infinite Intent is: The infusion of frequency to disintegrate static patterns of old beliefs and worldviews.

∞

*Shevevech sihutbaha minuvich heres arasta prihubat skrihus plava irechvi haranas, istetvravi misenech harasta briharavash uhunu-asta paravit.*

An increase in light will cause a new song to sing in the frequencies of our lives; this too will set us free from the old patterns that have kept us captive.

*Chevevech manesh hustel vavaa pra-unit herstaa. Privet archba sparet hurahes travaa ninuhet archba neshvi ehere nusvastaa prihuket arek pli-uhes arsta urahet ustechvi virspataa.*

The manifestation of thoughts and fantasy occurs because they are emphasizing certain equations within the One Life. All possible equations already exist; our focus brings them into experience.

∞

*Kirch eres erastu klihurava hereste unas perehur arek viret spa-uha viraset mispa kleherenek. Sutva pri husetvi etrek bispahur miravit brivek vrahet biritretvi anunas. Krihuves brihat virebrechvi harunas vastat erekta mishet uherenanuvis uvispata.*

Each person is the equivalent of a living library of possibilities. The possibilities are activated through eons of experience and held in the body and bodily fields of man. It is important to live beyond the possibilities inherited from the past by expressing from the timelessness of our being.

PART III

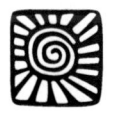

# Related Insights from the Tablets of Gobekli Tepe Secrets of the Whale Libraries

# Secrets of the Whale Libraries
## Secret 1 - Eating

- Despise not your humanness as an unworthy vehicle of eternal expression. The functions of the body have sacred messages from the timeless expression of your being.
- Eat in silence, for the act of eating is a sacred communion with the natural kingdoms. Through appreciation are you both fed by this experience. The plant and animal kingdoms thrive through being appreciated.
- If the flesh of animals is eaten, the bowels need to be washed.[1] The toxic waste products of meat will else linger in the intestines for many years. This irrigation of the bowels needs to take place every 7 days, if meat is consumed daily.
- Like the plucking of a string of a musical instrument causes other instruments' strings in the vicinity to tremble in resonant sympathy, so too food affects you. It provides a note that causes certain notes within you to vibrate in a sympathetic response. This is the way nutrition stimulates fullness of expression that produces health.

**Note**: This is also the way homeopathy works.

---

1 Enemas do not reach deeply enough. Colonics are far more effective.

Many remember the time of innocence when individuated life began and eating was not necessary, for resonance between beings served the same purpose of reminding one another of songs that needed to be sung. As life explored density, more notes became unsung and the ability to hear the notes of inspiration became lessened. Food became a way to stimulate unsung songs.

- The preferred way to eat is with your hands as metal utensils disturb the song of the food. (Homeopathic remedies should also not come in contact with metal.) If metal is used, let the handles be of the wood of trees. Let your ploughs be of copper; your pots be ceramic.
- Eat not standing up or lying down, nor when in stress, that the stomach be receptive to receive the food. Lie not immediately after eating, but if you must, let it be on your right side.
- Eat in silence as far as possible, that the communion with your food be deep and powerful. Pause in gratitude for the life you are ingesting, that the benefits may be increased one hundred fold. Eat your largest meal when the sun is high, and eat not after the sun has sunk below the horizon, that your body may rest in peace.
- Let your body become a grounding rod on Earth by balancing your food and sitting on the ground every day. The neutral charge of such a one averts catastrophes and helps all in his environment flourish.
- Many seek to return to a self-sovereign state of having no need for sustenance. Freedom from the need for food can only come to the surrendered life, in which the Infinite Song of Existence sings through your being. Only when you are authentically expressing shall you be free. Most avoid acknowledging the fullness of the present because they are so occupied by the past.

*Secrets of the Whale Libraries*

- We second-guess the fullness of the moment through judgment, thinking that something is lacking or imperfect. There is no failure – we have whatever is needed to contribute to the fullness of the moment. Judgment of what is lacking, or the illusion that the outcome could be failure, is born of blindness. A grass stalk blowing in the wind cannot see that its movement is not just haphazard. From above, the sweeping dance of the field of grass, as it is stroked by the wind, can be seen in huge moving patterns. We lack the perspective of the grand scheme of things because of the limited ability of the egoic self to see.

***Note**: By 'balanced' diet to assist a neutral charge in the body, the records are referring to a balanced ph (alkaline/acid ratio) in the body. Too much starch or meat for instance would create an acid body, prone to disease.*

*The records also specify the time required for either sitting or walking barefoot on the ground, as 'the time the sun would move the distance of two fingers, held at arm's length, through the sky. That is roughly an hour or 45 minutes per day. Sitting on concrete would also work.*

*Secrets of the Whale Libraries*

## Secret 2 - Sacred Sexuality and Relationship

- Many programs there are, given by the tyrants of man, that deliberately create guilt of sexuality and shame of the body. The power of sexuality is so great that were it known, the tyrants would be tyrants no more.
- All beings have their magic, but man has lost his way. The magic of man can be restored by remembering the potency of sexuality, and by evolving his concept of the expression and purpose of sexuality.
- Like the iceberg that lies mostly beneath the ocean, the true sexuality of humanity is largely unexpressed. When aspects are unexpressed, our eyes see life by what it lacks, rather than what it is. The more of ourselves we express, the more we are pleasantly amazed by what we encounter on our never-ending journey of existence.
- The feminine within all, holds the poetic perspective. See yourself through the eyes of the poet, for only then can you see another the same. Adorn your bodies and faces. Let your clothing reflect the song you wish to sing with your day rather than hide or shape the parts of your body you do not find acceptable. The body and clothing, and other adornments you may choose, are the joint poetic expression of your being.
- Sexuality is the holy communion within the temple of self-discovery you call relationship. Relationship is ignited by the spark of romantic attraction, but then tends to dwindle in its magical intensity. The linear progression of occurrences redefines it in ever-diminishing ways the more we label and think we know our partners. Like a sound that echoes back and forth, in decreasing magnitude, between a canyon's walls, is the linear progression of a relationship.

- Think not you know another, for their vastness is beyond your comprehension. If their responses are predictable, they have been captured by the imagined prison bars of belief systems. The evolved sexual interaction with your partner can liberate through the depth of the experience.
- The gift of deeply aware sexuality is to change the linear progression of life, which results in aging or the dwindling of romance into mediocrity. Change comes like a series of starbursts that shatter the prisons of existing paradigms, rather than like a fading echo.
- Have no agenda, nor expected outcome, but the joyous communion of the real touching the real with your partner, for within each dwells that which is timeless presence. The desire for outcome stifles life's spontaneous song. From expectation comes linear mediocrity. From spontaneity comes orgasmic starbursts.
- The core grief of man is the inequity and discrepancy in how much is given and how little is received. Deep, evolved sexuality flushes up core griefs long buried, creating fear that when one expresses in fullness, the other may spiral into volatile insanity. But when the real beginningless core of one, seeks out the real in another, the dross of the past rises and is consumed by the fire and blows away like ashes in the wind. In this way, change is leveraged beyond linear change.
- In mutual sexual surrender, man's obsession to know can be released as two become one. The songs yet unsung within each can be awakened. The song of innocent trust in playful adventure can take the place of planned strategy. The song of childlike wonderment at experiential discoveries of the self, takes the place of the obsession to know.

- Take time to enter the beauty of another and allow the other access to yours by lowering your shields. Then shall your true essence meet that of another. Know that you each are a portal into infinity, through which you may enter with reverence. Then shall the pure notes of your being resonate in a fluid, harmonious symphony. You shall find, in the timeless moments of your union, that the outer and inner have become one, as you ricochet with each breath between the depths of your partner and yourself.
- Know the rapture of the orgasms of the body by knowing the orgasms of the soul. The intense appreciation of another's potency and attraction can be called gratitude – the core origin of an evolved physical orgasm. Deep love and inclusiveness is the origin of the peak experience known as an emotional climax. The latter can be experienced with another, or with an experience of oneness with nature or art.
- The third form of orgasm is of the spirit. It arises from peak states of praise and is often referred to as rapture. The body, soul and spirit are unreal vehicles of our experiences as we pass through life, death and ascension. These three types of orgasm burst the boundaries of their grip of illusion on our reality.
- Sing now with your lives, the song of complete self-expression, that it may be remembered that these three mirrors that form the matrices of existence, have never been separated. Then shall the indivisible, timeless form, that has had no beginning, lift you beyond the treadmill of the illusional journey of life, death and ascension, to the miracle of eternal, ever-renewed form.
- When sexuality is denied as unworthy or unholy, sexual tension is often redirected into activity. This increases electricity in the body, making sexual expression more mechanical and perfunctory, while reducing the magic sexuality can bring.

- When the balanced, grounded polarity that evolved sexuality can bring is not present, the hyper-electric charge of the body calls in catastrophic change rather than graceful transition. A balanced polarity creates of a person a grounding rod that helps the seeds of potential in others to flourish. We stimulate fullness of expression in others, by living it ourselves.

*Chevevech nesetuch hurasvavi menevash asti kravis.*
Authentic expression eliminates mirrored divisions.

*Keresech prihas nanasvi uresta blavabit eres kerenat spihur mesenech krihavi.*
The sense of adventure stimulates open receptivity to the wonder of self-discovery.

*Prihas usetve minach usevi krivanut plihavas krives erech eseta mesenech uset harasvi.*
Contracted and shallow perspectives destroy the poetic perspective necessary for refined expression.

*Secrets of the Whale Libraries*

# An Example of the Glyphs from the Libraries of the Two Whale Libraries

### (The Story of the Ancient Ones)

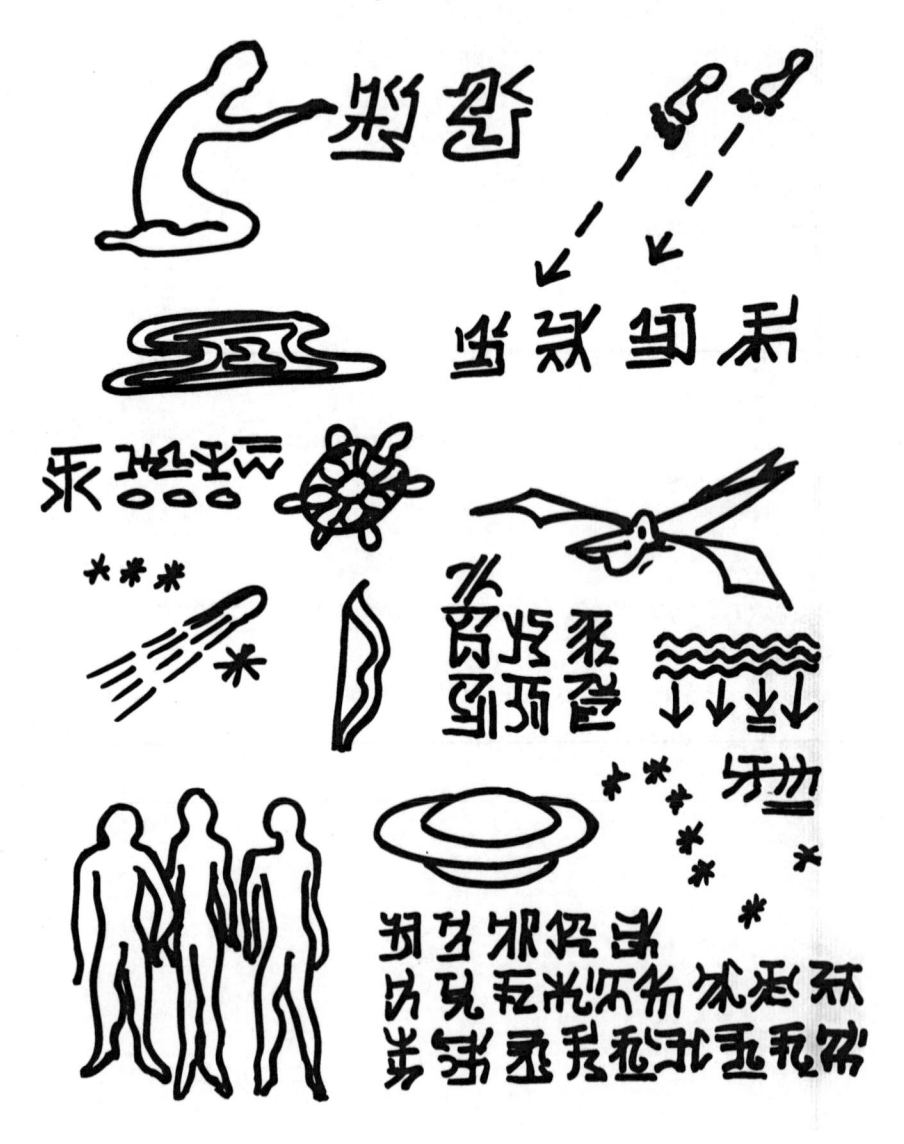

80

# Secret 3 - Abundant and Authentic Living

*Kishat ararech minetvi huraras kilechba husanet echparurarek esetvi manunach petreve skluharu-bat.*
Innocence is not blindness, but comes from deeper vision that sees the eternal within the heart of illusion.


- Our core fears seek resolution and obstruct the effortless flow of the divine expressing through us. A prominent fear is lack of abundance. Abundance is enhanced by praise and gratitude. Praise is an exalted state of being that lives above appearances and acknowledges the fullness of the moment.
- Soul, body and spirit are the vehicles of illusion that are formed from the stories and identities of the past. They deliberately create trigger events that bring back issues from the past in order to strengthen their existence, by our repeating those former events. As we become aware of events influencing us from the past, view them briefly from a perspective of yourself as vast as the cosmos, then shift your focus to the fullness of the moment. Like the stalk of grass blowing in the wind, know the perfection of the large picture manifesting through its parts, even if it cannot be seen.
- What then can the desires of your heart seek that is not already there? What prayers can you offer to heal the imagined lack of the moment? The desires that you feel are but the stirrings that awaken the unfolding notes of the Song of the Self.
- The folly of others has been a source of fear – those who in a lower reality dwell – for they seem to be the many and you are but one. Could they not bring the cloak of density and its consequences into your reality? Know now with compassion, that

the misbehavior of another is but an expression of their eternal luminosity reaching for its place upon the imagined stage of existence.
- The reality of each being is a unique slice of existence, and in that slice which contains all representations of the whole, he is the sovereign point of origin. When he is at one with the expression of the whole, his reality will be one of grace. When he closes himself to the gentle whisperings of his eternal being, and tries to impose his agenda onto his environment, his world becomes a cage in which he must wrestle with the demons of his own fear. Another's reality cannot affect him – two different slices are they. All that he can ever know is that all that is in his slice of reality can be affected by him.
- The world we know must change as we do, for within the spaceless space of eternity, we dwell within all and all dwells within us. We are not limited by numbers, since division is but an imaginary tool of the poetic expression of our being. Release now the fear that your endeavors cannot have the significant impact you intend.
- The guidance we seek from within or without, affirms relationship and strengthens division. The mirrors of the external exist also in the internal when we differentiate between the inner and outer. We are the portal of spacelessness; seek not the answers without or within but let the emotional nuances within and subtle currents without, guide your attitudes. From these shall the qualities of the day, through the attitude they evoke, steer the inevitable and right action of your life.

- From the food that you choose or the sexual images that arise, you are reminded of the songs you have forgotten. To the aware they stimulate the emotions and the attitudes that are dormant, to bring new expression to your life. View nutrition not as a need but an inspiration.
- The mirrors of body, soul and spirit have become the identities we think we are. But they are the garments we clothe ourselves in, for like all garments, they are a means to artistic expression, fashioned from the stories we have created. When we think that our form will perish if we discard them, we hold onto them until they become our armor. But the fluid form we are has eternally been.
- True eternal form is beyond the matter you know. It is that which has worn matter like a garment. Within eternal form, soul and spirit are aspects inseparably expressing as one with matter. There are belief systems that cast the separate shadows of the divided expressions of body, soul and spirit.

The separating beliefs are:
1) That the realm of soul promises freedom after death from the constrictions of physicality. Soul promises freedom but does not allow individuality of expression.
2) False values have been placed on the levels of soul (death) and spirit (ascension). They are thought to be more holy, merciful and knowing than the physical.
3) The physical has been seen to be more mundane and mediocre. But to the one that is aware, its stark contrasts (causing the tension that maintains its density) offer the most exquisite poetry and deepest rapture.

*Secrets of the Whale Libraries*

- Abundance is the triumph over the illusion of limitation, the song of power over appearances. Refuse to accept programs of negativity. Minimize lack by shifting the focus: envision the opposite of what you fear. Live abundantly in your own reality and all else shall flourish.

*Bereshpa mishet harusta misech haras erestatve*
There is no adversity, only reminders of unsung songs

## I AM

I am the thunderous clamor
Of one thousand pounding drums,
Heralding to an astounded world
The eternal glory of the rising sun.

I am the elusive, unfathomable silent wonder
Of a rose unfurling the mantle of its velvet petals
In the heart of the night.

I am the ever-receding depth of darkness of the starry sky,
Offering its shrine to the shining celestial jewels
Of the still whispering constellations.

I am the wild laughter of the thunder,
And the burning embrace of the lightning,
Piercing the sky in an outburst of joy
Across a summer storm.

Eternal mystery am I,
Revealing myself through riddles
Throughout the fabric of time and space,
Relentlessly weaving ever-changing scenes
On the dreamed canvas of my existence.

Marc, Belgium

## Secret 4 - The Nature of Change

- The nature of change can be either cataclysmic, or a graceful metamorphosis from one level of existence to another. Cataclysmic change comes from the surface and forces us into re-evaluation and the eventual adjustment of core beliefs.
- Graceful change is precipitated by a deep and profound shift of core attitudes and beliefs. This foundational adjustment filters into the surface experiences of everyday life, resulting in graceful and supported change.
- The future is written in the moment in the same way that the past is fluidly reformed by a well-lived moment. If we abandon the moment by fearing or anticipating the future, we forfeit the priceless gift of the power of the moment. We lose the ability to not only determine the quality of our existence, but the way in which change will occur – with grace or cataclysmically.
- We are standing on the cusp of a deep core shift in cosmic and planetary existence. This will most certainly filter through into the surface conditions of everyday life. Whether we experience these changes with grace or trauma depends on how fluidly we can synchronize our deep, inner change with the profound and fundamental changes taking place at the heart of existence.
- We have been part of linear change as a way of life for eons of existence – this is about to change. Linear change causes deterioration in all circumstances, unless we constantly feed it energy to maintain ideal conditions. This principle is called inertia.
- The peak condition of the body, or a relationship for instance, deteriorates without constant efforts of renewal. Linear change is like an echo bouncing off canyon walls – it becomes weaker

every time it changes direction. The canyon walls can be equated to cataclysmic change that forces life into a different direction. Cataclysms cause shock, and shock lowers consciousness by creating a loss of life-force and energy.
- The way life changes from one expression to the next throughout the cosmos will become a starburst rather than a line bouncing off the membranes or matrices of space.
- The movement of life within a confined space is the experience of liner time. The space is formed by limiting belief systems that confine our experiences within matrices.
- The effect of exponential starburst changes at the heart of life is the shattering of layers of matrices. This changes not only the way time will be experienced, but also effects instant freedom from old belief systems.
- Previously changes came from cataclysms and opposition (the canyon walls). The result was deterioration in the quality of life. The changes at the heart of existence will now come from rapture, and will release profound energy and life-force (supported change) to the surface conditions of everyday life.
- As the cosmos transcends the principle of inertia, one of the core griefs of man can be healed: the belief that our output (effort) always exceeds our input (rewards). It is now possible to flourish and to achieve results more effortlessly – embrace this belief. Replace doubt with glad expectations. Repeat the daily affirmation: I flourish by releasing old expectations.
- As the gap between cause and effect closes, thoughts and feelings will more rapidly manifest. Be aware of your fears, but immediately redirect your attention to their opposite manifestation: If you fear lack of resources, acknowledge your fear but immediately pour energy into the visualization of abundance coming into your

life until what you fear seems unreal. Do not pretend negative emotions are not present as one strengthens what one opposes, but rather withhold your energy from them by redirecting it elsewhere.
- Live with deep awareness. Slow life down and take a few pauses in your daily activities to appreciate deeply your environment, others, your many blessings and the Earth. Gratitude brings increase and self-appreciation. By allowing yourself to be inspired by your environment, your life becomes revitalized.
- Attuning to the unfolding core of existence through gratitude, love and praise, creates peak orgasmic experiences of the body (sexuality with the self or another), the soul (emotional rapture such as that inspired by art, music or deep love) and the spirit (through praise resulting from the recognition of the perfection unfolding beyond the appearances). These create starburst experiences that shatter old matrices and birth new possibilities.

# Secret 5 - Nuances of Eternal Expression

Ten fears are there, that cause victimization. Ten feelings that move with silent power from our eternal core, that when expressed, can remove these fears. Self-pity becomes replaced by the fullness of our eternal song.

## The Fears of Victimization

1) Fear of victimization from authority
2) Fear of the folly of others
3) Fear of the tyranny of the body
4) Fear of the dictatorship of the soul
5) Fear of the control of the spirit
6) Fear of ancestral programs and heritage
7) Fear of insurmountable opposition
8) Fear of annihilation (not being worthy of life)
9) Fear of not being prepared or adequate (performance angst)
10) Fear of being unsupported

## Nuances of Eternal Expression

1) Timeless self-sovereignty – Living from outside the matrix one can direct, through slight intent, the experience within the matrix.
2) Receptive expression – Receiving inspiration from the world around us allows our expression to be aligned with unfolding existence.
3) Full appreciation through an omniperspective – We cannot find the inspiration from our environment by just using our eyes or ears alone. Allow yourself to absorb the eternal

aspect of what you observe, feeling it through the inner as well as outer senses.
4) Exponential discoveries – Change linear becoming to starburst, exponential becoming by leaving the past stories behind. Discard all identities. Allow the rapture of deep experience to shatter the shields of shallow vision.
5) Inspired Oneness – In seeing the beauty at the heart of all life, we awaken it in our own, through resonance.
6) Unconditional love in response to recognition of beauty – Love evoked by inspiration is unconditional and without agenda. This transcends one of the biggest obstacles of the heart: Loving without pain.
7) Truth as spontaneous expression of your eternal being – Truth cannot be sought, but needs to express as the free, pure spontaneity of your eternal self.
8) Awakening the eternal song by finding astonishing wonderment everywhere – We change our reality by seeking the poetry of our existence. By being aware of brutal circumstances, but choosing to focus on the praiseworthy, we empower a higher reality, benefitting all life.
9) Revitalizing communion with the timeless aspects in all things, through aware acknowledgment – Decay occurs by focusing on the imperfection of appearances. Life is revitalized by living from core to core through awareness.
10) Exchanging the mirrored existence for authentic expression – The five senses alone provide false information and trick us into thinking we know. A life of authentic expression acknowledges that since life is forever new, nothing can be known. The truth of the moment must be felt.

# Closing

Amidst the abundant outpouring of revelations and sacred tools that have been provided by the Seer Almine during more than a decade, the Yogas of Illumination have been some of the most instrumental in profoundly benefitting lives around the world.

Her revelations and translations of ancient records range from the deeply metaphysical to the practical application of the mystical concepts. The yoga practices given in Aranash Suba Yoga transform the practitioner at the non-cognitive core of the psyche – the pivotal level to facilitate graceful and effortless change.

*May the blessings this Yoga of Enlightenment can deliver, find fertile soil in hearts of receptive humility. May the unfathomable discoveries of the self, as an aspect of the One Life, reveal themselves on our never-ending journey throughout eternity. It is my sincere prayer, that as the light-bearers of the planet, we may see with childlike eyes of wonderment, the ever-unfolding truths of this great adventure of existence.*

*To the Infinite the glory, forever and ever.*

Almine

**Related products by Almine**

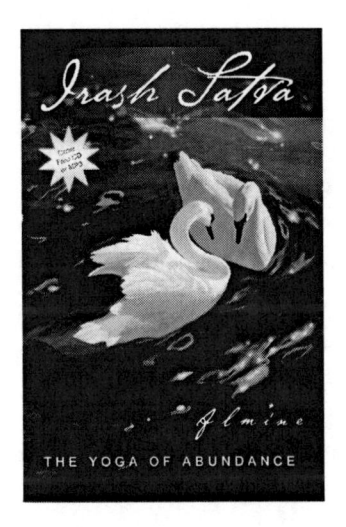

## Irash Satva Yoga
**The Yoga of Abundance**

Yoga, as a spiritual and physical discipline has been practiced in many variations by masters and novices for countless years and is universally accepted as one of the most effective development tools ever created.

Man's physical form in its original state was meant to be self-purifying, self-regenerating and self-transfiguring. Through pristine living and total surrender, it was possible to open gates in the body that would allow life to permeate and flow through it; indefinitely sustaining it.

In Irash Satva Yoga, received by Almine from the Angelic Kingdom, this ancient methodology is exponentially expanded and enhanced by incorporating the alchemies of sound and frequency.

Using easily mastered postures paired with music from Cosmic Sources created specifically for each, the 144 cardinal gates in the mind and body are opened and cleansed of their dross and debris, allowing the practitioner to tap into the abundance of the One Life. Includes MP3 download of the 24 Sound Elixirs of Hidden Kingdoms plus Klanavik I and Klanavik II.

Published: 2010, 94 pages, soft cover, 6 x 9, ISBN: 978-1-934070-95-3

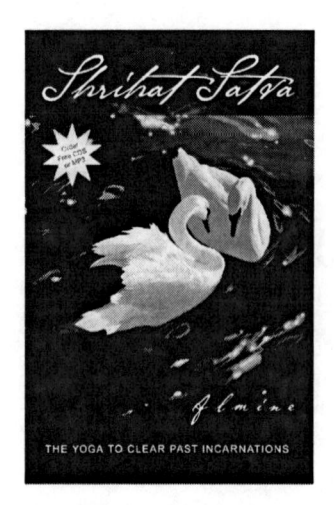

## Shrihat Satva Yoga
**Yoga to Clear Past Reincarnations**

The human body is unique in that it is an exact microcosm of the macrocosm of created life. There are 12 points along the right, masculine side of the body and the same number on the left side. These are microcosmic replicas of the macrocosmic cycles of life.

The yoga postures are designed to open and remove the debris from these points — the gates of dreaming. This will occur physically through the postures and the music. Dissolving debris also occurs by way of dreaming (triggered by the breathing and eye movements), releasing past issues that caused the blockages in the points.

Includes the 24 Sound Elixirs for Freedom from the Dream and the Poetry of Dreaming Pre-meditation as a 2 hour MP3 audio download.

Published 2010, 108 pages, soft cover, 6 x 9, ISBN: 978-1-934070-15-4

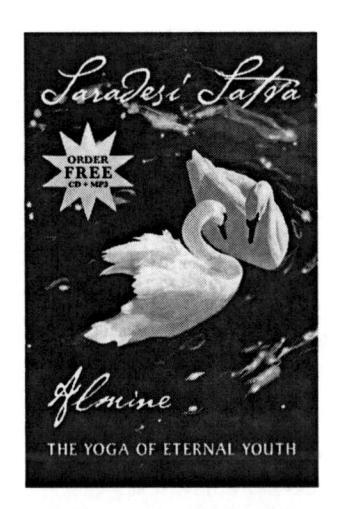

## Saradesi Satva Yoga
**The Yoga of Eternal Youth**

    As translated from the ancient texts of Saradesi – The Fountain of Youth. The ancient texts speak of time as movement. They affirm that time and space, movement and stillness, are illusions. To sustain any illusion requires an enormous amount of resources. This depletion of resources causes aging and decay. The illusion of polarity, the impossibility that the One Life can be divided and split is brought to resolution by balancing the opposite poles exactly. Only then can they cancel one another out, revealing an incorruptible reality that lies beyond – the reality of Eternal Youth.

Published 2011, 115 pages, soft cover, 6 x 9, ISBN: 978-1-936926-05-3

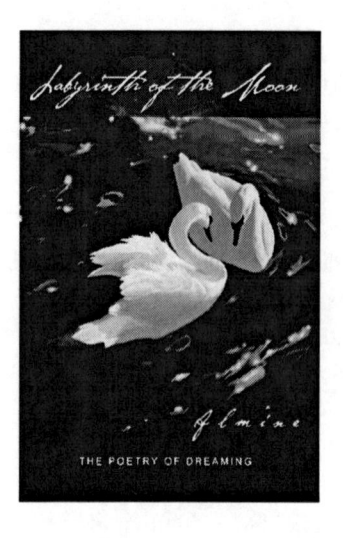

## Labyrinth of the Moon
**The Poetry of Dreaming**

    This book contains 144 verses of the Poetry of Dreaming and extensive lists of the interpretations of dream symbols. It is a valuable tool for opening up the deeper dream states' communications, promoting the healing of the psyche and the body as well as facilitating the balance of the Inner Child and other sub-personalities.

    Designed to release the hold of past incarnational cycles, it is an essential companion for practitioners of Shrihat Satva Yoga, but also a great book just on its own.

Published: 2010, 239 pages, 6 x 9, ISBN: 978-1-934070-10-9

---

Visit Almine's website www.spiritualjourneys.com for worldwide retreat locations and dates, online courses, radio shows and more. Order one of Almine's many books, CD's or instant downloads.

US toll-free phone 1-877-552-5646